It'll Happen By 30

A Relentless Journey of Faith
Delayed But Not Denied

Marline C. Duroseau

ROYSTON
Publishing

BK Royston Publishing
P. O. Box 4321
Jeffersonville, IN 47131
502-802-5385
http://www.bkroystonpublishing.com
bkroystonpublishing@gmail.com

Cover Design: Elite Book Covers
Cover Photo: @Photosbyreem Kareem Virgo of Reem Photography
Additional Credits for Photoshoot for Front and Back Cover
Planned by: @nerievents
Styled by: @simplytiffannie
Makeup: @picaasso
Hair Styled by: @nickimarshal69

ISBN-13: 978-1-951941-99-4
LCCN: 2021916423

King James Version Scriptural Text – Public Domain

Printed in the United States of America

Dedication

This book is dedicated to all the women and couples who are on a quest to start a family and it didn't happen in the time or way they planned. It takes perseverance to struggle and push through in spite of the trials, tribulations and disappointments. I hope my story and experience will help provide comfort and hope to the readers in a similar situation

This book is also dedicated to all the Angel Babies in Heaven. They have made the ultimate sacrifice in the name of their families. Not having you around is not and never will be a tolerable experience in the lives of your parents. I pray you continue to watch over those of us still on this Earth going thru the journey. You are remembered and celebrated daily and especially on your birthday and National Pregnancy and Infant Loss Remembrance Day – October 15.

We love and miss you always Angel Grace Duroseau. Thank you for your sacrifice. Gone but never forgotten ~ 12.21.2011

Acknowledgements

Thank you to the Lord, my God, for EVERYTHING. Without his love, grace and mercy, neither myself or my family would have this story to tell. Thank you Lord!

A huge thank you to my mom, Isilia Louisseus and dad, Barthol Cepoudi. Thank you for giving me life. Thank you for teaching me to love the Lord with all my heart so that he may grant all my heart's desires. Thank you for teaching me to never give up and never settle for anything less than greatness as I work towards accomplishing my goals. A special thank you to my mom for being my role model. Mom, you have shown me how to love my children unconditionally while also reminding me to never lose myself in the process. You are my hero - I love you mom!

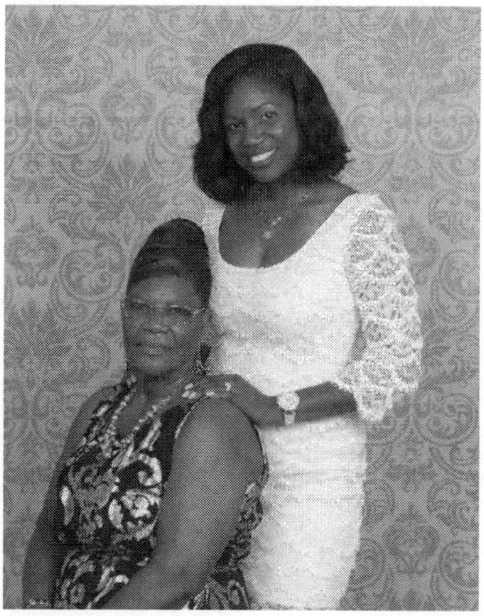

April 15, 2016 – Our 35th & 70th Birthday Shoot: JCPenney Portraits

To my husband Kevens. You are my rock and biggest supporter. Thank you for being my best friend in allowing me to be the different versions of myself. Thank you for providing unconditional love and support as I navigated these many levels of my life. Thank you for being and staying on this roller coaster with me. Thank you for never making me feel like I am less than a woman because of the path we had to embark on to have our family. Thank you for being a wonderful husband, reliable and superhero dad to all of our children! We love you and thank you!

Thank you to all of the boys' aunts and uncles, their God-parents, honorary God-parents and my extended work family who are also the boys' aunties. Thank you for all your supportive efforts and love before, during and now after the struggle!

I cannot leave out my cousins, especially Laurie Joasil and Charlene Labranche. You ladies have no idea the love and gratitude I have in my heart for you. Thank you for all your planning, running around, sleepless nights, phone calls, prayers and most importantly – the unconditional love and support before during and after for each experience. Love you forever. Thank you.

More specifically, a thank you to my in-laws, more aptly referred to as in-loves:

My husband's mom, Raymonde Telfort, you came into my life literally at the most perfect time. I am not sure where I would be on this daily mommy journey without you. Your patience, love, sacrifice and determination to help us raise these boys is beyond anything I could ever imagine. Thank you for loving the boys and making sure they are cared for day in and day out. You are our light and we pray you continue to shine with us daily. I love you.

Ulrick and Nela Duroseau, my husband's dad and step-mom – Thank you for helping guide us on this journey to conceive. Thank you for your advice, love and support before, during and after our quest to start a family. I am forever grateful for how you accepted me as your own since day 1. As such, my problems became your problems and you fought alongside us as we searched for solutions. For that, I love you always.

Choubert Telfort and Nezie Delima, my husband's brother and sister. What more can I say? If I call, you come, if I text, you come, if you even think the boys need you, you magically appear. No questions asked. Whether near or far you're there. Sad days, happy days, you're there. I am not sure how I would be able to maintain any sense of sanity if it weren't for your unconditional love and support, especially as it relates to the boys.

Thank you for Everything. I love and appreciate you more than you'd ever know.

To Margaret Fernandez and Mary Anne Wood my mentors, turned friends, turned family - I could not have accomplished any of this and more without you both! Thank you and I love you!

Thank you to the members of the group You Are Not Alone (YANA) and its founder Manouchka Valcin. Thank you for serving as a major source of support, a familiar outlet, a Christ-fearing group of people that truly served the purpose of providing help, support and mentorship for each other. Being a part of YANA played a significant role in my life during the 'trying' years. I am forever grateful and blessed to still have the friendships we formed over 13 years ago.

Thank you to all of my siblings – Bertolet Cepoudy, Yveline Cepoudy, Kedlaire Augustin, Sudney Cepoudy, Wilkens Cepoudy, Emma Arnett and Berny Cepoudi. It's amazing how we all have a new bond to share – parenting. I love seeing the future through the eyes of all of our babies. Through the ups and downs, I could always count on all of you to be there. You always showed up in support. That means the world to me. Love you all.

To my big sister Yveline, the mother of my first born kids – Thank you. Because of you, I think I know what I am doing with my crew of boys. Thank you for letting me love your babies like my own because for a very long time, they were all I had. Thank you for being an excellent role model in exhibiting true super mom values.

This book is also dedicated to the selfless medical staff that assist and care for Reproductive Endocrinology, Infertility, Prenatal and Postpartum patients. To all the Doctors, Nurses, Acupuncture Doctors, Therapists, OBGYNs, MFMs, Radiologists, Pharmacists, Phlebotomists, Embryologists, Surgical technicians, Anesthesiologists, Medical Assistants, everyone essential to the cause but often go unrecognized – this is a dedication to you. I hope this book shows you what a light you are in the lives of so many of us and the impact you have on our individual journeys.

Thank you Dr. David I Hoffman and entire staff at IVF FL Margate. What more can I say? We've been thru the trenches together and I am happy to say - we won! I am not sure where we would be without your dedication to helping Kevens and I realize our dream. I am forever grateful. You are truly a light of hope and inspiration to so many, like myself, that find themselves in a world of despair and uncertainty.

Thank you Dr. Farrar Duro and staff of Florida Complete Wellness. The use and incorporation of acupuncture in conjunction with fertility treatments while trying to conceive proved to be a recipe for success in my case. Having acupuncture before, during and after each and every treatment cycle and pregnancy helped me in more ways than you know. You helped fix a lot of my problems - bleeding, swelling, cycle quality and overall tranquility. I am happy I found you Dr. Duro.

Thank you Dr. Salih Yasin, Dr. Gene Burkett with the University of Miami / Jackson Memorial / Holtz Children's Hospital & NICU for caring for me during both my twin and singleton pregnancies. You helped save both my life and that of my boys. Thank you for equipping me with the confidence I needed to get through these pregnancies on the side of success. You are amazing.

Thank you to Julia Royston because I found out about you at the right time. Even after having our initial talks about getting the book done, you gave me the space I needed to get my life back on track after having our last baby boy. Throughout those two years, from initially reaching out to actually working on the book, I kept hearing in my head "Let's go," and I was finally ready to pick it back up again. Since then, we've been non-stop in trying to get this book done. You motivated me to get it done and helped me be OK with telling MY story openly and freely. You also helped me see how my experience will be an inspiration to and help many others to come! THANK YOU!

Definitions

TTC – Trying to Conceive	Menopur – Fertility Medication	ET – Embryo Transfer
IUI – Intrauterine Insemination	Follistim Fertility Medication	DPT / dpt – (#) days past transfer
IVF – InVitro Fertilization	Lupron – Medication used in Fertility Cycle	3dt – 3 Day Embryo Transfer
TAC – TransAbodominal Cerclage	Crinone – Progesterone Medication	5dt – 5 Day Embryo Transfer
NICU – Neonatal Intensive Care Unit	BCP – Birth Control Pill DH – Dear Husband	(#)wk (#) d – # weeks and days in pregnancy
HCG – Human Chorionic Gonadotropin	PCOS – Polycystic Ovarian Syndrome	5wk3d = 5 weeks and 3days pregnant
E2 – Estradiol (Estrogen Level) Estrace – Estrogen Pill	FET – Frozen Embryo Transfer	OBGYN – Obstetrican Gynecologist (Pregnancy Doc)
PGS – PreImplantation Genetic Screening	ERA – Endometrial Receptivity Analysis	OB/MFM – Maternal Fetal Medicine (Hi-Risk Pregnancy Doc)

Table of Contents

Introduction

What is a plan? A plan is a detailed proposal for doing or achieving something. When someone plans, they are deciding on or arranging something in advance. Everyone has a plan. We plan for how we'll get through school. We plan for a milestone trip and celebration. We plan out the week to see to it the weekend is used for something in particular. We plan our routes when traveling.

In essence, it is a good idea to have a plan, right? Unfortunately, life would not live up to all it's cracked out to be if everything went according to plan. It is inevitable that some plans may not unravel as intended. When this happens. This is where the multitude of tests come in to play. The tests of faith, the tests of reliance, the tests of loyalty, the tests of patience, the tests of endurance and perseverance.

As I provide the detailed steps of my and my family's infertility journey, you will experience and witness along with me the unplanned series of events. I would like to add this was my experience. Everyone may not experience the exact same thing and your journey may be different. One thing remains constant, there is a lot to unpack on this trip and hopefully my story can help sift through all those layers without falling apart.

Contact Info –
Email: info@happenbook.com
Instagram: @itllhappenbook
Website: www.happenbook.com

It'll Happen by 30

So tell me, have you always wanted kids?

Yes. This is a loaded question that has been asked of me time and time again. Ever since I was small, I might have been 10 yrs old and I just knew I wanted kids because I come from a big family. So I wanted the same thing, 10 kids to be exact. My mom and dad, Barthol and Isilia, have five kids together: My sister, Yveline, and I and three brothers, Sudney, Wilkens and Berny. My dad has three additional kids, Bertholet, Kedlaire and Emma. So there's eight of us. My dad comes from a large family as well. There were a lot of siblings — there might've been seven or eight of them. My mom's story is a little sad. I know her mom passed away when she was nine. They both went to bed and fell sleep together, and when my mom woke up, her mom was not awake next to her. I also know she was the baby of her family. She always talked about her older sister and I think one or two brothers, maybe there were about four or five. I'm not really sure.

So, I never met my grandmother. I always wondered what my grandmother was like. As a matter of fact, I didn't get a chance to meet either grandmother, and it's indeed sad whenever I think of it. So I cherish the relationship I see day in and day out between grandparents and their grandbabies. It's a different level and type of love.

By the time I became a teenager, I still wanted children, but I definitely didn't want 10 anymore. I lowered my count. I'm like, Oh, I love the kids because I used to always be around my cousins. There were a lot of us and we grew up together. Although there were eight of us kids, all of us didn't grow up together. My little brother and I were born here, and then I had two brothers and sister come from Haiti when I was nine.

So we went from having only a four-person household that all of a sudden grew to seven. They were five kids and I was nine. So my brother and I, when you're nine, all you know is American life. You don't know another language. My dad spoke English. My mom didn't speak English that well, but we communicated — she's my mom. Like it wasn't an issue, you know? So now I'm nine and I had three more siblings who just came here, and we're trying to each learn each other's language to communicate. And then by the time I turned 15, another brother came. Also, in the middle of all of this, I have a sister who's Bahamian. So we knew her too, and even remember some visits and interactions but she didn't live with us.

Then my final brother, Kedlaire, lived in Haiti; he didn't come to visit until I was about 16. He is a lawyer. He came to America for some kind of law school international program.

All throughout my adolescent years, obviously I wasn't thinking about kids. I was a straight A student. I was just focused on school, hanging out with my friends, you know, getting along with my family, just doing that type of thing. So I really wasn't worried about it. At that point, that was when it was the “say no to drugs” era and “no teenage pregnancy” era. No one was thinking about having children at that point.

I was helping taking care of kids from the age of nine, like my cousins, neighbors and things like that. So I've always been around little children. Then my sister started having kids because she was a little older than me. When I was 12, almost 13, she had my first niece, Beatrice. So, we were like sisters, you know? So then she had another baby, Brittney, and another baby, Brillana. So between being like an older teenager and a college student, I was also helping take care of my sister’s children. I really enjoyed spending time with and helping care for them.

Then at that point, I met my husband, and we weren't thinking about kids or anything, but we were together since I was about 16, 17. I moved out when I was 18, which was really young. Now that I look back on it, I know why parents worried and do what they do because you think you're grown.

You think you are, but you're not, you're not.

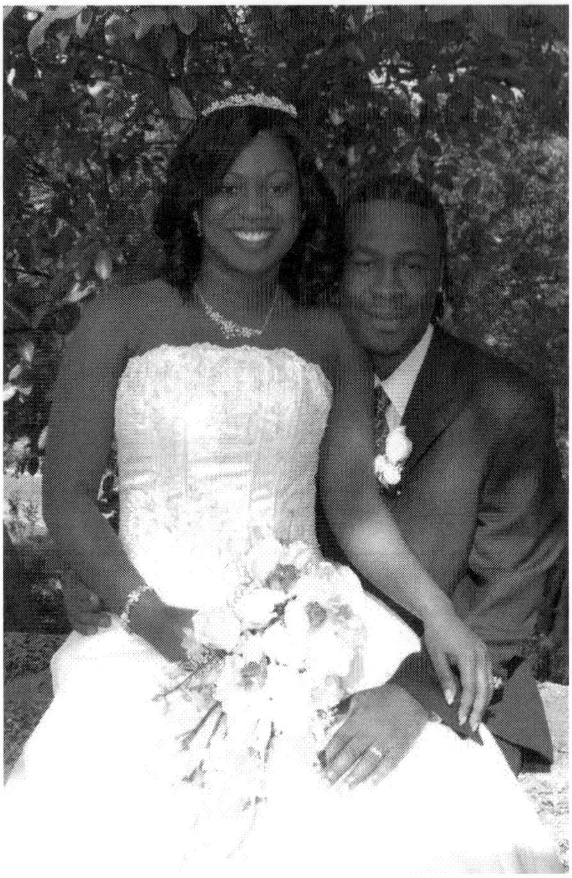

(Feb 2008 – Josue Photography - wedding pictures photo reshoot)

It's Time to Start the Work - Let's Get Checked Out

I moved out at 18 and we got married when I was 21. At that point having babies just wasn't happening, but it was OK because I was still in college pursuing my bachelor's degree. So when I got to be around 22, 23, I said, you know, I need, we need to go get checked out to figure out what's going on because you know, not that we necessarily wanted it to happen, but there were no accidents. Like nothing was going on. And at that point my husband already had a son, Richard. When I met my husband, his son was one, almost two. He was his only kid. So in the Island community, I figured they just automatically assumed that, Oh, you know, he has children. So he's not the problem. I thought everyone felt it was obvious, it should be me. It's what my thought pattern was. No one really asked us our plans or talked about it. It came up sometime but not often. My husband was a good sport. I was about 23 when we started to look into going to the doctor, and I remember there was this nice Jamaican lady at a doctor's office, Dr. Mark Goodman, I went to and she's like, "OK, why are you guys here? You guys are young. It just takes time. It'll happen." I said, listen, don't tell me I'm too young because then I will be 38 and then you're going to ask me why didn't I come when I was younger. The lady starts laughing and she says, "You know what? You're right. I never thought about it like that." So, and then we ended up staying with that doctor, Dr. Mark Goodman. You know, when you go to someplace seeking whatever help, regardless of what it is, you feel hopeful and ready to be like, "Oh, OK, it's going to work."

My marriage was strong. I was finished with school. We were trying to buy a house. Like everything was falling in line the way it should have, but it still never happened. We had a few treatments with Dr. Goodman. We had three cycles of intrauterine insemination (IUI), not the invasive in vitro fertilization (IVF) yet. But for IUI to work, you need a really strong sperm count.

With IUI, they bypass the vagina and just put the sperm in the uterus and it is less distance for them to swim. Each time we went to do it, the sperm count wasn't there, you know, something was going on, but they didn't necessarily say anything was wrong with me. So we're all looking at each other, like how come he has this child but yet the sperm numbers just aren't there now? So, all of a sudden there's an issue, you know, on his side. Around this time, I started to hear the office throw around the term PCOS (Polycystic Ovarian Syndrome) as maybe something I might have after going through all of my diagnostic screenings. So after those failed three cycles, we eventually switched doctors. It's about five years later. In that meantime, we bought the house. I went back to school for my Master's Degree. We renewed our vows and had a church ceremony and huge wedding. It was important to me to get married in church as I felt that just made our union more official, if that makes sense, in front of the Lord. It was a beautiful celebration! I was also trying to get my CPA license. So, I just had other things to occupy my mind. In the meantime, my friends were having kids.

My sister had another baby, Ysvelt my 1st nephew, too and everybody around me was married and having kids. I can also say I was a proud auntie and god mom to many of the babies. I didn't let it bother me too much, but it impacts you, you know. I never had a jealous or envious feeling in my heart. And I know it's really important for people to know that because the one time I did, I literally lost it. I finally had that moment in January 2010 where I was like, "Woe is me." I was depressed. I cried. I was upset. I said, "This doesn't make any sense. This is just horrible." And then my husband goes, "It's OK. It's OK to let it out. You know, you're not a bad person because you feel that way." You know, why me? Why, why, why?

It Should Happen By 30

So back to 2003, we had had those treatments that didn't work. We took a little bit of a break. I had other stuff going on, explained above. And then in 2008, 5 years later, we went to see Dr. Kenneth Gelman. He too, did some diagnostic screenings on me and found some of the indications of PCOS. I don't remember Dr. Gelman being or showing much of a concern about my levels or polycystic ovaries as my body did what it was supposed to each month and my hormones, although borderline, was not out of whack. We did an IUI cycle with clomid and then another IUI cycle with injectables, higher doses of fertility medications. I always responded well to the medications. Those treatments didn't work, either. I remember going during lunch for one of the IUIs and Dr. Gelman was just shocked. He even suggested we cancel the transfer because the sperm count and motility were both so low. I was devastated. I did it anyway but all in all it resulted in a negative pregnancy test both times. I remember him telling me, things like, "You need to relax, go and take up yoga, do some acupuncture, try to relax, don't be as stressed out about it because even if you don't feel physically stressed, subconsciously it's manifesting and it's 'gonna impede whatever it is you're trying to do."

Also in 2008, my childhood friend Sonia invited me to join a support group, YANA, which stands for "You Are Not Alone!" The group was created by a young lady, Manouchka, who wanted to bring young married women and couples together who had experienced miscarriage, loss, infertility, etc. It truly was a breath of fresh air. As many of us were from Island backgrounds and educated professionals, yet we shared that common feeling of having these taboo issues plague us in one way or another. There weren't many people we could talk to. Having this group was just great.

My first meeting was very memorable and therapeutic, as well. You think you have a tough time and then you find out others have experienced the same as you. You also find out others are in much more difficult situations than you. It was a very eye-opening and humbling experience. I love the group and its members.

Upon speaking with one of the ladies and deciding on next steps with fertility plans, I found out about a company that offered refunds if you did not take a live baby home. My pursuit of that option is what led me to Dr. David Hoffman and IVF FL (IVF Florida)! So at that point, I did take up yoga in 2009 after both Dr. Gelman and Dr. Hoffman recommended I do so. I loved it. I started Bikram Yoga, one of the toughest because it's conducted in a hot room. During my consult and subsequent work-ups with Dr. Hoffman, we found out I needed a surgery for something. So I did that, and everything turned out fine. I needed to have a hysteroscopy and laparoscopy procedure. It turned out it was just a blood clot that looked like something else on a diagnostic screening ultrasound.

As explained, it was my uterine lining that hadn't shed totally after my period. So they weren't sure if it was a polyp or fibroid. I mean, so at that point, you're thinking, OK, now you really want to think maybe that's why it didn't happen because this was what's going on. So we did that surgery in 2009, everything ended up fine. It was just some blood that needed to be cleaned out. So that was perfect. Dr. Hoffman also found as a result of my diagnostic screenings he was not totally convinced I have a PCOS diagnosis. He could agree I had some of the individual symptoms relating to PCOS, like the excessive facial hair, literal ovaries that were cystic and filled with follicles even when not stimulated, borderline testosterone levels, etc. However, all else did not lead to that as a finite diagnosis, especially because I menstruated each month and my hormones during the different stages in the monthly cycle adjusted accordingly. As we would find, my body responded extremely well to any medications I was given. Thus, he felt even if it were PCOS, it was not really an issue – it could be addressed. He agreed with Kevens and I moving on to IVF and thought we'd be successful because of the process's evolution to kind of bypass the sperm count issue, reducing the large number needed.

Throughout this entire time, my husband was working overnight. And when I say overnight, I mean he started work around five in the evening and didn't get off again until five in the morning.

It takes a toll on you, the relationship and your plans. As time went on, I decided to start planning my 30th birthday party. I said to myself, no, it's time. This is my focus. I have my Master's, I just got my CPA license, we have a house, we have great jobs. We have everything. I told my husband, "We need to work on changing your schedule so we can focus on having these kids." I really felt this is the year it's going to happen; I just knew it. I just kept saying to myself, this is the year it's going to happen. So, surgery in 2009, mental breakdown where I felt jealousy and was update in 2010, then the big 3-0 to come in 2011. I remember like it was yesterday.

And I said, "Yes, this is when it's going to happen. You need to change your schedule because you need to be with me. We're going to have these kids. And I don't want to feel like a single mother." He said, "Single mother?" I said, "If you're working overnight, when you come home, you'll be asleep. So who's going to help me with the children? I'm not doing that." You know? My husband was able to work on his schedule but the change did not last long. He eventually was offered more money and a promotion to return to the overnight shift because it was just not going well without him.

At this point, we would be given a blessing in disguise in that his mother was to come from Haiti. His mother lived in Haiti this whole time. The plan was she was going to live with her daughter because her daughter had like seven kids, five biological children of her own and then two more from her husband. So there was more of a need to help her with the kids. So, you see we both come from large families.

It just so happened my mother-in-law ended up wanting to and staying with my husband and I. And she's been with me ever since. Thank God, because I don't know what I would do without this her. Yeah.

She came to America for the first time the day of my 30th birthday party. She arrived in the morning of April 2nd and the party was that evening.

Did I Meet My Goal?

Let's go back a bit more. After meeting Dr. Hoffman in 2009 and then having the surgery, two years just kind of flew by. I actually did not move to the next steps right away because we were holding out hope that things may just happen naturally since having the surgery. That had been the experience of many others – where they have the exploratory surgery that in a way helps clear things up in there, and then they fall pregnant shortly thereafter. Unfortunately, that was not the case for us. It's now February 2011 and I was almost 30, just a couple months shy of the big milestone birthday. I was at a crossroads of sorts when it came to work during this time. By now, I had been with the company for nine years. I had my CPA license and was offered a job at another company in January 2011. It was a difficult decision to determine whether I'd leave or stay. All in all, I decided to remain with my company. Although challenging, I felt it was the right place for me because of my history and tenure there. Besides, if we wanted to start a family, I figured I'd stay where I can be afforded flexibility because of my tenure and relationships with my managers. It was tough because the regulatory agency that governed our industry mandated all reporting be submitted and up to date. Failure to do so would result in a $5,000 fine for each report that was still outstanding. At the time, we needed to have 11 of them filed. So, it definitely was a trying time. I was able to get them all done by the April 30, 2011 deadline, all while planning and having my 30th birthday party as well!

I then became physically and mentally exhausted. I literally shut down. I needed a break. My manager was anticipating that day would come and kept offering for me to take some time off but I kept saying, "No, I'm OK" and then I wasn't. Needless to say, I took about three weeks off after having filed all those reports. It was much needed. I also used that time off to focus and reassess what we wanted to do next.

We decided it was time to seriously start trying again: full steam ahead with IVF. We contacted Dr. Hoffman and started cycling in late May 2011, the month after my 30th birthday and meeting that huge work deadline! When I returned to work after taking that time off and agreeing to start cycling, I had a conversation with my manager and HR director explaining what I was going to be embarking on. They were very, very supportive. My manager felt confident in knowing I could juggle all the work responsibility and medical appointments. My HR director had gone through this process before, so she was a great friend and resource to me when it came to coaching me through the process or just being supportive.

Cycles normally take up a two-month period. Our actual retrieval and transfer cycle happened in July 2011. That's when I became pregnant for the first time ever. The first time I did IVF, I said, "Well, we're going to go with a package," because back then they had multi-cycle packages. In case it didn't work, you can try it again without having to spend all that money. So at that point I said, "It'll be our luck. We pick a three-cycle package and I bet you, I get pregnant on the first try."

The Calm Before the Storm

We didn't even make use of the money spent on the multi-cycle package. So yes, we got pregnant the first time. It was exciting. Everything was going great. There were no issues with the pregnancy at all.

And then all of a sudden, everything was not fine. I was almost five months along. I didn't have any pain. I didn't feel anything. Everything was fine. I went to the restroom and I passed what looked like a clot. I said, "OK, well, this doesn't make any sense." So I called the doctor, and the doctor said, "Oh no, come right over."

I went to the doctor's office and when I got there, I was on a high. I was like, "I get to see the baby on ultrasound! Yeah. I walked in to the office with "How are you doing? Oh, your dress is cute." I was just oblivious. I had no idea what was to come.

So my OBGYN, Dr. Marion Lacombe, was in the ultrasound room and she and the ultrasound technician were talking. Between the doctor and the ultrasound tech, they were like, "Oh, do you see it?" And I was like, "Yeah, I'm looking." And I didn't see anything because by then I had already had 10 years of experience with ultrasounds. I know what things look like on the ultrasound. I didn't see anything. So I was not worried. I was not in pain. You know, everything was fine.

So then the doctor came in and she said, "Well, let me pull out an image for you." So she pulled out an anatomy prop thing. It was a 2D or 3D image of the uterus, the vagina, and the cervix. She said, "Well, this is what your uterus looks like. This is where the baby is. This part here is supposed to be closed. And yours is open one centimeter." I said, "Excuse me?"

And she said, “Yes. So in essence, the baby could just come right out if this is not closed.” I didn’t know what that meant.

“Do you know what happened? How do we fix it? What's going on?” So in essence, I never ended up going back home. They called my husband and he drove to the hospital. The doctor said, “Well, we have to have surgery to try to sew it closed.” The problem was, they didn't know how long it had been open. So the regular bacteria in the vaginal canal probably got in there. They wanted to hurry up so that they could close my cervix, as they didn’t want to shut something and then trap the bacteria in.

We didn’t know how long it had been like that because I had no symptoms. You know, I had no discharge, no nothing, no pain, nothing at all. So to make a long story short, we did the surgery, the surgery was a success in that after you are cleaned up as best as possible, they sew up the cervix with the placement of a cerclage.

The plan was I was going to stay in the hospital on IV for about a few days just to monitor and make sure everything was OK. Then I would go home and continue my life with my cerclage in place. These strong stitches were there to help you carry the baby to term; then they take the stitches out when it’s time to deliver.

I remember being in recovery and then the monitors just kept going off because I kept having contractions, whereas I wasn't having contractions before. They didn't hurt, but they were being picked up on the machine. So they're like, you know, we're going to keep you here longer so that we can monitor and try to stop these contractions.

They ended up giving me magnesium, which messes up all your muscles. So it's like your body is like flailing, no strength, no tone, nothing. Like you have no say, no control. It's horrible, that drug, but it stopped the contractions. They told me OK, you're 20 weeks and we're going to try to get you to 24 weeks. Once you're 24 weeks, that's viability, the baby has a 60% chance to survive.

So in my head, I'm going, “OK, well this is a first. I didn't know it. OK. Well, thank God we found out now because we're going to figure it all out and I'm just going to go on about my business and continue my pregnancy. Now we're trying to see if my kid will have a 60% chance of surviving?” It was mind boggling.

Time to Brace Myself

I ended up being in the hospital for a couple of weeks. One day I didn't feel good; nothing hurt, but I didn't feel good. I just felt weak and felt feverish; I just didn't feel quite right. But in the meantime, they were doing urine tests routinely to make sure I didn’t have a UTI. They took my blood to make sure I didn’t have an infection. They were doing all of this a couple of times a day. And then one day, I remember it was a Sunday, we were watching football. I'm a football fan. We were watching the game or something like that. I then had a few of my friends and family came to visit because more people are off on the weekends. So they came to visit. And then all of a sudden I said, “You know, I need a towel on my head because my eyes felt heavy.” And my husband's like, "You don't really look too good." I said, "You know, I don't really feel too good. I just feel very tired." And you know, it was as if everything steamrolled at that point, the nurses came in, they're like, "Oh, you know, your white blood cells are a little elevated."

Mind you, I've been lying in that bed now for two weeks because every time it seemed as though it was getting better, something came up and it was like, "Oh, let me watch you a little more."

Then I got better then I wasn't. In the meantime, they didn't want to touch my cervix, but technically they had to check it to make sure it's not open. So I was also having ultrasounds done to make sure that the cervix wasn't opening silently again. It had been going on two weeks at this point. I didn't feel good.

So they gave me Tylenol, which helped the fever go down. But then Monday I ended up feeling bad again. And that's when everything went to hell. My blood work came back really bad. I went from my having a minimal elevated white blood cells to, "All my blood is bad and they need to get the baby out, and I'm going to die and this pregnancy needs to stop now!"

So at that point, the infectious disease doctor came in. The NICU (Neonatal Intensive Care Unit) doctors came in and talked to me because by now I was only 21 weeks and six days, almost 22 weeks. So they ended up saying that there was nothing else they could do if they didn't deliver the baby, because I had a severe life-threatening blood infection now. So if they didn't deliver the baby, I was 'gonna die and all this other stuff.

They explained they would do their best to try to see what they could do for the baby and yada, yada, yada. I remember it was 3 p.m. They said, "We'll give you the medication to start labor at 3." They wanted to do it at 3, but shift change was going to happen at 3:30. So between 3:30 and 4, I got the first dose of labor-inducing medicine. And do you know of all things? My epidural didn't work. They give me the medicine to start the labor. OK, great. I was in labor. Fine. I was like, OK, I'm going to get an epidural. The epidural didn't work. And when I say "work," I mean, like you get stuck with the injection in your back. And it's supposed to numb you. That didn't happen.

This was my first time, so I didn't know the feeling. My sister had never had an epidural, either. At least with me, she's always been natural and just taken her IV meds and that's it. You know? So the epidural doesn't work and I was like, "my belly is not numb, I feel the cramps because if you take the belly as a circle, and then you put it in quadrants, the part up here was numb." "The bottom two quadrants were not numb." The cramps felt like somebody was slicing me with a knife. It was horrible. And so they gave me more medicine and then another part became numb. So I was numb in 3 of 4 quadrants, but I was still feeling the contractions and pain. So they gave me more medicine. And at that point, I think that's what did me in because now instead of the epidural numbing me from the belly down, do you know it started going up? So now I was freaking out. So I couldn't feel myself breathe.

Of course only like 1% of the population ever, if that, gets that effect. So I said, "I don't feel good. I feel like I'm about to die. I can't feel myself breathe and dah, dah, dah, gibberish." So they had to stop the epidural, and that last quadrant still wasn't numb. And in the meantime, the nurses and the doctor were checking and they were like, they didn't need me to dilate that much because the baby would not be that big. So, you know, they were kind of watching it.

In the meantime, my room was full of people. My poor husband. Let me tell you about this guy. He was there the whole time, but he was on the bed that's in the room, laid out like a corpse covered with the sheets and a pillow over his head. And he's just like that in that position the whole time I'm in labor. I'm like, "What about my husband? What about him? Is he breathing? Can y'all check?" And my mom, his mom, his step-mom, his dad, his brother, my sister, my niece, the room had like 17 people — God! So I'm like, "Can you guys check on him?" And in between me wanting to see if I could breathe, I was checking on him.

And he told me, "No, I'm fine. Just focus. I wish I can hold your hand." I said, "No, you stay right there." I know he's very squeamish and doesn't like that stuff or hospital settings at all. It's crazy because this would be the first of many more hospital stays to come and he braved up to the max for those.

He Giveth and Taketh Away

So I remember the nurse came in and she goes, “Okay, mom, I'm going to check you.” And she checked me and she said, “OK, you're about six centimeters. You can start pushing. Let me get the doctor.” She called the doctor in.

Then the doctor came in. And you know, it's funny because she had a French last name, but she never spoke Creole. The doctor was a young to maybe late 30s-aged lady, very sweet lady. I noticed her last name was French, but we never spoke Creole. There was no reason to.

So I remember she came in and she said, “All right, baby, it’s time.” And she asked, “What are we going to do?” And she's like whispering to me while she's down there. And she said, “Well, what about all these people in the room?” And she asked, “What do you want to do?” I said, “I don't have a problem with them being there. I just don't want anybody in my vagina.” And she started laughing in understanding.

My mom-in law who was sitting directly across from me and had a blank stare in to the direction of my legs. Remember was still new to America, and I had just started to establish a relationship with her because she came in April. I got pregnant in July/Aug cycle and now we're in December. It's been a little bit, a few months. So the doctor turned around, and she said in Creole — first time I ever heard her speak the language — and she said, “Mommy, can you sit over on this side? I don't think it's good to have anybody directly in front of her." And my mother-in-law went, "OK." And everybody just looked up and surprised because we never knew, you know, you don't want to assume, but it was so nice that she did it in her native language. So they had her move away and she just said, "Okay." The doctor then said to my mom-in-law, "I can give you a job. You come hold this leg." My sister was holding the other leg. My mom was standing by my head at the top of the bed. The whole time I was in labor, I just remember singing. Yes, Jesus loves me. You know, it's taking me back, but I sang that the whole time.

I asked my brother-in-law to take pictures, but not to look at my vagina. It was so funny. Everybody starts laughing. They're like, "Well, how is he to do that?"

My father-in-law was off on the cot with his son, my husband. They were just praying, you know, things like that. And then I ended up pushing the baby. I think I pushed three close back to back pushes. She came out, and it was horrible. It was horrible. I was afraid to open my eyes. I didn't want to look at her. It was as if I was shy and afraid. She had like a shocked look when she came out. It was like, "What's going on? Where am I?" Like, that's how I felt her breath was. And then that was it. She was gone. Like I just knew, you know? So she took those two breaths or a breath and a half, and then she was gone.

And then finally, and I felt like the light, it was all of a sudden, a blinding light that was so bright. And I had my rosary with me. After she came out and I was able to open my eyes, I looked at her and I was like, “Oh my gosh.” She looked just like her dad, my husband. Her body resembled that of my brothers Berny and Wilkens. They both are tall and skinny. And she had that exact same shoulder clavicle frame. And I couldn’t believe this was like an actual little human. She was perfect in her skin.

Everybody was taking pictures, everybody was crying. And then I told my husband, I said, “I really think you need to see her because I think you'll regret it down the line, if you don't, you know?” And he said, “Oh, I get it, I'm just too afraid. I don't want to.” I said, “No, no, no, don't worry. You have to come. She doesn't look bad. Yes. She passed away. But she doesn't look bad. She was like a brand new born baby.” He ended up looking, and later down the line, he said, “Thank God you had me look because I couldn’t just imagine what the baby would look like forever versus actually seeing her for myself.”

So, we named her Angel Grace.

I had made friends with the housekeepers, and it was so cute because they had come in and were like, “Oh my God, I'm so sorry.” One of them left her prayer card. And then the dietary lady, the one who brings the food, she had come in earlier and she was like, “Oh, I know you like Frosted Flakes. So I'm leaving those for you now.” Yeah. I had Angel Grace after 13 hours of labor. So I must have had her at 2:53am or 3:53am, like that next morning. So the shift had changed. The overnight staff let the early seven o'clock staff know what happened. We had called the priest, Fr. Kiddy, over, but he was unable to make it in time to bless or baptize her. He was able to visit me the Sunday, two days, before I had her and had said a prayer for her and us.

The hospital had a chaplain who came and said a prayer with us. She was with us for a good little bit. We took pictures and then finally they had to take her away. We have to, you know, fill out forms for a death certificate, and tell our intention for funeral plans, etc.

I Don't Have my Baby but my Body Did

At that point — remember I'm on the maternity floor — and then I got really sick. I got really sick. It was as if my body was poisoned. I spiked a fever after I pushed out the baby. My sister was still with me; everybody else had left. Then all of a sudden I couldn't control my bowels. I felt like this rush of, of whatever it is, come over me.

It was like poop started coming from my head like a river and then everything came out. I was so embarrassed. I started crying because I was embarrassed, but all the nurses were like, "No, no that's OK. You should start feeling nauseous. Let me go get you a bucket." And I was like, no, I felt —, and then the minute I was going to say, "fine," the nurse came right in time with the bucket. I was throwing up green stuff above and diarrhea at the bottom. It was fast and they weren't prepared. So they couldn't even put chucks under me because they had already cleaned me up from the regular delivery. It was horrible. Horrible. And it was very humbling, too. In that time, I found time to write this beautiful message to Angel. I remember having my Blackberry, and I typed it up and sent out notifications to my family and friends of her birth and death.

So then at that point the doctor said, “We're going to move you from this floor because although when you're in your suite, you don't hear other people having babies....” So that was very sweet of her. I didn't even think of that. She said, “We're going to move you.”

So they moved me to a regular floor, and I had the nicest nurses. I remember waking up in the middle of the night screaming in so much pain that I had to press the button. And then I was like, “My chest hurts. My chest hurts. Something's going on!” And they were like, “No, my dear, that's your milk coming in.”

Well, it came in with a vengeance. It was as if somebody took cement rocks and just threw them at my boobs. It woke me up in my sleep in the middle of the night. I had never had a baby before.

I couldn't leave the hospital until the Infectious Disease doctor released me. I had something like five bacteria in my blood that they had to clear out of my blood stream before I could go because I had become septic. So at that point, I said, “Listen, I don't know what you're going to do, but you need to clear me before Christmas because I can't be in this hospital on Christmas day. Like you you're just going to kill me. I'm just going to die. You know?” He said, “No, no, no, but you have to feel better. But I promise you we'll get you there.”

No Baby No Visitors – Leave Me (I Want To Be Alone)

On the bright side, the Infectious Disease Doctor discharged me and I was told I'd be going home the evening of Christmas Eve, I believe. Of course, this news came with a double-edged set of emotions. On one end, I was happy to be leaving that horrible reminder of hell. On the other end, leaving meant I would have to face the fact that I no longer had my baby growing inside of me. Even worse, she was no longer even alive. I could imagine that the ride home would cut so deep. As we drove east on Miramar Parkway to get home, the sun was glaring. Instead of serving as a sign of a bright future to look forward to, the rays of the hot sun felt as though I was being blinded, burned and stabbed over and over again. I couldn't escape it. I cried and cried as I reflected on my time at the hospital. Now that I was heading home, I could only think of the royal purple box I was given in the hospital. I guess it was to serve as a keepsake to remember my experience, my first born, my Angel. I know I keep using the word horrible but that's just what all of this was...horrible. What was in the purple box? Well, there were2 pictures of Angel, official foot and handprints – they were so tiny and perfect, a card containing her biological info – height, weight, name, birthdate, etc., a memorial card, her hat/bonnet and a tiny outfit or wrap of some sort. That was all I had to remember her as the days went by.

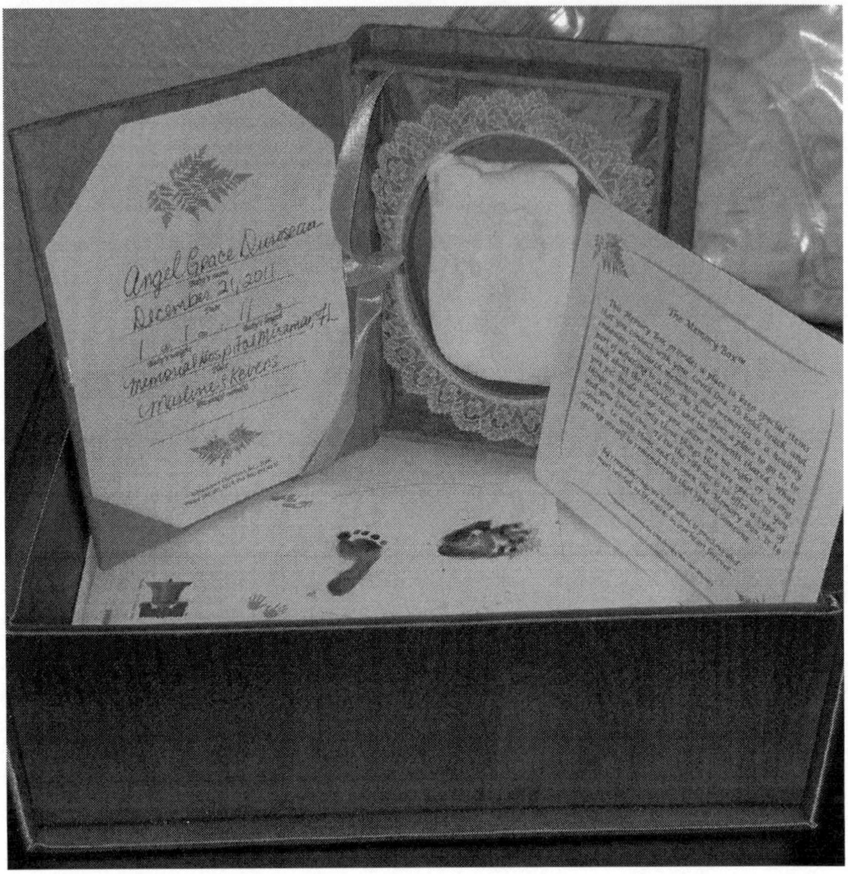

(Dec 2011 - The “Purple Box” – Keepsake box given at hospital after delivering baby Angel)

To make matters worse, for me, when I got to the house, everybody was there. My husband's son was there for the weekend. I am not sure he knew what had happened but I didn't want to see him or my husband’s cousin, like everybody, my family, etc. At the end of it all, I feel it was really tough and I didn't want to see people. So imagine coming home from the hospital, and the house was full of people. I didn't think to say or inform my husband, “Don't have anyone there.” I just thought he’d know. In the Haitian culture, being there and showing up was their way of showing support.

I just wanted to go in my room and shut the door. The people brought me gifts and different things that I was very appreciative of. I just didn’t have the mental capacity or wasn't in the mental state to talk to anyone because I did not want to be borderline rude.

Especially the older generation, they don't realize what they're telling you because I guess they were raised to just act like, OK, that happens. It happens to everybody, so it’s normal. It is then that I found out how many of them had had that same experience, but no one talks about it. They'll say, “Oh, that happened to me. I had to deliver three stillborn kids or I had....” And I was like, wait, what?!?!

So at that point I was intrigued on the one hand, because I was like, “Oh my gosh, like how did you deal with that?” And then on the other hand they're like, “Well you just put your big girl panties on. Babies will come again.” Literally, the saying is “babies come one behind another from the house headboard" or something. It's a literal translation. So I know it doesn't make sense, meaning right away I'd be pregnant again, so don't worry. I'd just have another kid because that's what happened to them. So in the meantime, don't cry. You can't be, you can't appear weak; just put your big girl panties on and just keep going. And I'm looking at them like you don't understand, like this was a life. Like she was moving. Like I felt hurt. There was a hole. And I said, "You know what? I can't."

It was hard. But I had two other friends who were the sweetest in the sense that they visited and they just sat with me. We were together for two hours. They said nothing.

That's exactly what I needed, because some people come over and they think they need to just tell you stuff. However, what they're saying either makes you upset or it makes no sense. I have to be respectful and listen because that's how I was raised, right. I had to sit there and visit with them when they came.

At one point I told my husband, "I don't want any more visitors," and I'll never forget how his best friend was taken aback and said, "Did you tell her it was me that wants to see her?" I felt bad. Like, "Why wouldn't she come out? Like, like she needs to see me. She needs to know I was here." He even had a beautifully wrapped fragrance gift for me. So the family is following the cultural tradition of physically visiting. They want me to see them so that I know they cared. I'm coming from, "I just need to be alone."" I don't think negatively of you because you didn't come in the room. It took a long time to go through things.

Therapy Here I Come

It was just an unbearable pain to bear, just horrible. So from that experience, I decided I had to do something because I was just not feeling better emotionally. I didn't think I'd go to therapy. I didn't know it would affect me as much as it did. My OBGYN set me up with a Therapist because when I went to see her for my one-month follow-up, and she was checking everything, making sure everything was OK, I was still crying. She said, "You know, this is very tough. I think you need somebody to talk to." She said, "Go and speak to someone and don't feel like you're being judged or feel bad, so you can express your feelings."

Again, it was horrible. Once I picked up the ashes, I finalized the funeral service with the Church. Fr. Kiddy performed a beautiful funeral mass for Angel. Many of our family and friends attended the funeral in support of my husband and myself. Their presence meant so much to me. The whole idea of having a funeral mass was hard for Kevens. After seeing how many people came out to support, it made him feel a bit better and less apprehensive about the whole thing. I felt he got to have closure after the funeral. I thought I would find closure as well after reading the poem I wrote for her to her at the mass. I must say closure did not and has not really happened quickly.

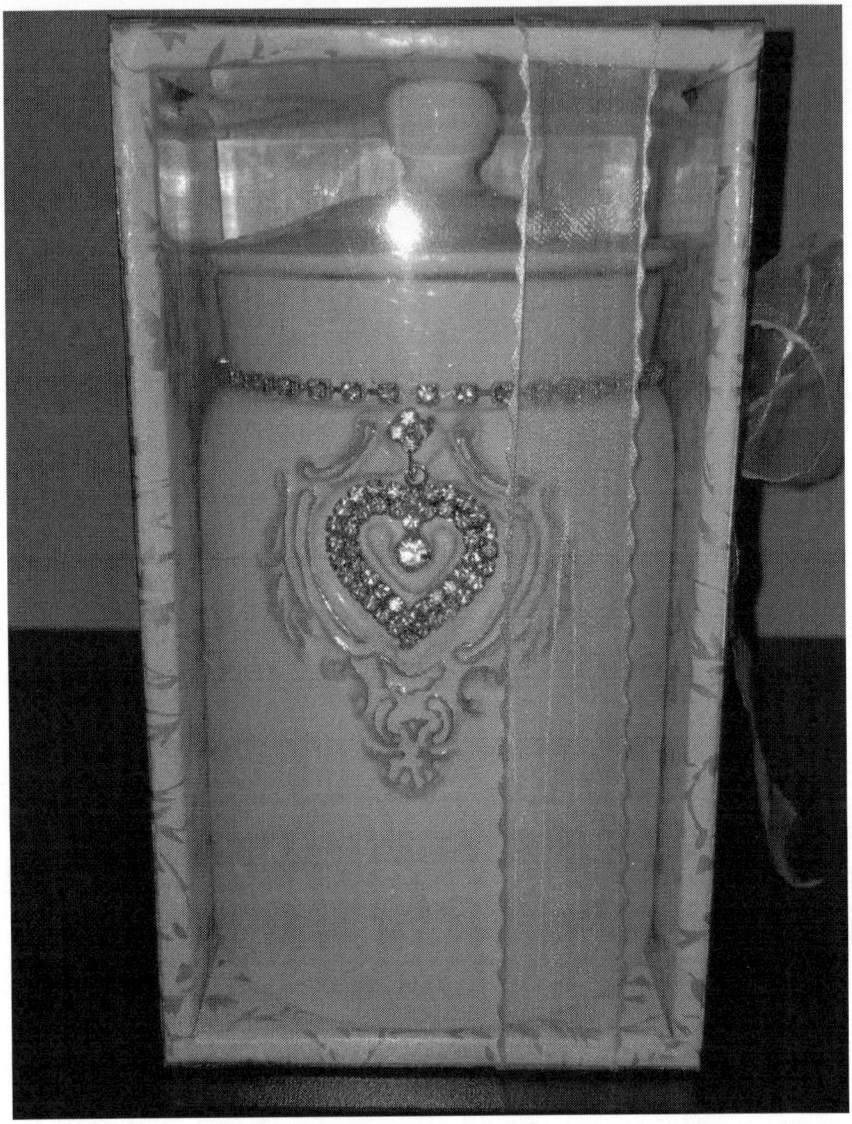

(Jan 2012 – Picked out this beautiful white urn for baby Angel's ashes. In remembrance of her and since the funeral, I wear white on Easter Sunday in her honor.)

Kev and I talked about what we were going to do with Angel's ashes after the funeral mass. We considered spreading her ashes out at sea. We also thought about laying her to rest in the cremation section of the cemetery. I could not and still have not been able to bring myself to getting rid of the ashes – they are still with me. As a compromise, I placed her ashes and the royal purple box in a place that's easily accessible and memorable to me but not as evident and "in your face" for Kev. After ensuring Angel was safely home with me, I was ready.

I was finally in therapy. I started two months after having delivered Angel. Dr. Gotthelf was like a God-send. There were some sessions where I just cried. During other sessions, I just sat and stared. I got to the point in therapy where I could talk about Angel and my experience without crying. Meaning, if I talked about her 10 times, I would cry now only seven times instead of all 10. My therapist was able to see the progress, too. I went to therapy 2x a week. We unpacked a lot of feelings. I just have to know that if I do get pregnant again, I'm going into it with the mindset of, 'yes, I'm still sad, but I'm also going to try to enjoy it,' I didn't want to go into it as if this chapter is done and now I need to live in this other chapter." And she said, "You know, you're one of the first patients to realize that trauma doesn't just leave you. You're able to move forward, but you're able to deal with knowing and recognizing that it's there, but you still have to try to move forward."

I knew Angel was with me the whole time and Dr. Gotthelf helped me come to realize her passing wasn't my fault. I wanted to try again right away. “OK. I have to go get pregnant now.” And then I said, no, because I felt it was my fault. “What if I did something wrong again?” So it took a while to get through those therapy sessions because even the doctors and everyone else say it wasn't my fault, I didn’t think that. So then I said to myself, “OK, what can I do differently this pregnancy to make that not happen?” And then it became, “OK, well, now that we know I have a weakened cervix, I'm going to go in and have a preventative cerclage at 12 weeks.” So therapy and intense researched made me feel I was prepared.

I had to be confident. My doctor even recommended me to the Jackson Hospital specialists and I ultimately changed doctors. There were no hard feelings. I still talk to Dr. Lacombe. She has three patients who are friends of mine that I sent to her because she's really good.

People at work were praying for me. So from December 2011 when I delivered to where we were at this point, realizing I was ready, was about five months post-partum. I went to my therapy session and I said, “You know Dr. G, I think I'm ready.

Let’s Try Again

I then contacted my IVFFL. They were like, “OK, Marline, it’s so good to hear from you.” In the midst of all of this, people were contacting me, checking up on me: the work friends, the staff that I made friends with at the IVF clinic, everybody. Thank goodness I had the multi-cycle package because the only thing I needed to pay for now were meds, which were about two to three thousand. The package that we paid for guaranteed you would come home with the baby within the three tries.

I had to get all the medical records from the hospital and forward the records to the clinic so they could update their program to reflect next steps. They needed to confirm there was not a living baby. I was able to start the process again without having to pay the entire IVF fee again. We felt very lucky.

Juggling Work, Life and Trying Again

After having suffered this devastating loss, it was clear, life doesn't just stop. I am still on the move at work! By now the company was growing, and fast. To go back a bit, I have always wanted to be a business professional. I work in the healthcare industry with Skilled Nursing facilities (SNFs). I've been with the same company since July 2002 when I was a senior in college. Then I graduated with my bachelor's in 2003. From there I just kept getting my education and receiving promotions.

I love it. I love the numbers. When I started, we owned only one facility but managed three. As time went by, which is what seems like each year, we acquired more and more facilities, causing my responsibilities to grow.

We acquired a new facility in late 2011, another in March 2012, and were in the works to get a new one in September 2012. That would bring the count to nine SNFs.

How do women do it all? Why was I just not able to plan when to get pregnant and have it just happen naturally — like what we see on television or in the story books? Well, I learned quickly that is not really how it goes down in the real world.

I was ripping and running with handling audits, daily operations, accounting staff and training under my boss, my mentor, the CFO. I found it a bit challenging to now have to worry about taking more time away from the grueling daily tasks and deadlines to make time for more appointments, tests, ultrasounds, etc. No matter what, I knew I had to do it ALL. I wasn't sure how I'd do it, but thank God for great staff, understanding management, a flexible work schedule, and a very supportive husband. All of these factors served in the right capacity because what we were in store for was so beyond unimaginable — a roller coaster of events and emotions. So, just like that, operation "Let's try again" began.

The Big Day

<u>Tuesday — 05.22.2012</u> — Today is one day before my next "big" appointment at the doctor's office. I am really hoping and praying that all goes well and falls in line with God's timing for this cycle so it can be a success. After work yesterday, I drove to Walgreen's Margate and picked up my meds. It took just a little longer than I expected due to a fraud alert with the Chase debit card, but after being on the phone with customer service for several minutes, we were able to get the transaction processed. I must also say that I broke down and purchased a small Blue Bell ice cream, cookies and cream, as they were on sale for two for $4.00. In an effort to not be AS bad, I purchased only one for $1.90.

In addition to that, my cycle started yesterday at around 5 p.m. I was not expecting it at all. Last year around this time, my cycle was a week late, meaning I had to wait a whole week to start my meds because at that time my E2 [estradiol] level would read low enough to start. So, to have my cycle start a couple of days early (basically on time), I think it may be a good sign that my E2 will come back within normal range allowing me to be able to start stims tomorrow night.

I am so anxious and ready for everything that I am finding it hard to really take things one day at a time. I am just really hopeful and prayerful for things to go well and that this cycle will be successful. I am willing do to everything as instructed by my physicians to ensure I don't mess things up. I have acupuncture tonight, and I am looking forward to that. I just find that I am in a much more relaxed state of mind after having the treatment. I also notice that my body functions a bit better, as well. Whatever ailments or uncomfortable feeling I have is gone after the treatment.

I am feeling a bit sluggish today, though. The Lupron is finally catching up to me. For the past two nights, I've experienced night sweats, and I think it's due to the hot flashes that are associated with taking the Lupron. I guess I'll have to ensure the a/c is on in the evenings so that I am not uncomfortable when I'm sleeping. Waking up to a soaked night gown and pillow is not a nice feeling.

Wednesday — 05.23.2012 — Ok, so today is a good day, thus far. I had to wake up very early, 6:15 a.m., not normal at all for me. But I made it to my 7:30 a.m. appt at 7:41 a.m. So, I didn't do too bad regarding time. Ms. Paula drew my blood. The u/s tech did the scan and said everything looked good. We counted 5 follies in one ovary and 7 in the other. In one of the ovaries, I had a small cyst. She didn't see reason for concern and thought the doctor wouldn't, either. I then met with Nurse Nadia. She is really nice. She went over the chart, how to administer the Menopur, how to work the Follistim pen, etc. Although I've done this before, I really needed the refresher to make sure I don't screw anything up :-/. She advised that I called phone tree to see what my blood, E2 levels, come back at. She didn't seem worried about the cyst, either, but said the E2 level is what will determine if we can proceed or not.

I arrived at work a little after 9:30 a.m. I checked phone tree at about 10:00 a.m. and no results yet. I then checked again at 10:30 a.m. or so and, yes, the results were there. Nadia was the nurse who left the message. E2 came in at 43.1, AFC [antral follicle count] is 12, and lining is nice and thin, perfect. She wanted me to consider again whether or not we were doing PGS [pre-implantation genetic screening] once the stims begin so that they can prep on their part. I then called the office and spoke with Nurse Adriana. She was nice, as well. I asked if the Counsyl genetic blood testing results were back yet. She checked the computer, and they hadn't been entered yet. So, she then logged on to the Counsyl website and, voila, the results are in. She happily told me that after going through over 300+ diseases and seven pages of results, I came back negative as a carrier of any disease tested that would result in genetic mutation! She seemed really pleased because she explains that normally people come back with something at least, even if very rare, but I was perfect! Thank you, God!! That's just one less thing to worry about.

I then asked her what she thought this meant in Dr. Hoffman's view regarding proceeding with the PGS. She explained that since everything came back OK with the Counsyl testing, she thinks he may continue to lean toward not doing the PGS on the embryos. We'll see how I respond to the stimulation meds, and he'll definitely make a determination then.

I'm feeling very happy about all the news and updates received today. Now I have to focus on administering my meds tonight, on time. Last night I totally forgot to take my Lupron. Thank God I called my husband once I settled in after the game, and he happened to ask if I took it and I immediately did so then ☺. I can't wait for him to wake up in a couple hours to share all of this great news with him. We're happy yet cautious and trying to take things one day at a time. OK, until later or tomorrow.

Thursday — 05.24.2012 — I'm having another good day today, thank God. Ok, so I told hubby about my appointment and calls with the nurse. He was excited to hear that all went well. I must say I had a long day and by the time I got home I was EXHAUSTED and sleepy. I just have so many things to do when I get home, that is part of my daily routine, which just takes up about another hour or so.

After making the bed, taking my shower, applying my medicated cream to my skin, etc., I decided to mix up the applesauce and probiotic and let it sit. Then I decided to prep up all my meds for the evening. There were three different syringes I had to prep for my injections. That took a while as I had to sift through all the Walgreen's bags and organize the meds and decide where to store them all. By now, it's like after 7:30 p.m. or so. I decided to administer my meds. I iced my injection site for a full five minutes. Whoever invented ice being used as an analgesic is a genius. It really helps take the edge off. I didn't feel any of the needles go in. When injecting the Menopur, it started to burn a bit so I had to kind of manipulate the skin and inject the meds slowly. Injecting the Follistim from the pen was easy breezy. By the time I got to the Lupron, I think I used a spot that wasn't as numb, so I had to ice for about another minute and then injected the Lupron. That was done. I noticed that I also bleed more from the Menopur needle so had to clean that up a bit. After giving myself all my meds, I had the applesauce and then ate dinner. I then felt like I had indigestion :-/. Next, I had to burn my moxa stick and do the treatments on my spleen points in my legs, another 20 minutes. It wasn't as bad, though, because I was watching "The Middle" on ABC. It was a funny episode, as usual ☺. After the moxa treatment, I began to struggle to stay awake. I was feeling very woozy and a bit sick to my stomach and very dizzy and lightheaded. I remember catching a little bit of "16 & pregnant" on MTV and that was it, I was out.

It's now morning. I was already awake prior to my alarm going off. But I still closed my eyes and said a thorough prayer while lying in the bed. As soon as my prayer was over, the alarm went off. I decided to prep all my meds before taking a shower. Once I prepped them, I figured I'd just administer them and go from there. I iced again for a full five minutes. I administered the Menopur first, as I figured I'd get the hardest one out of the way first. I didn't feel the needle going in but started to feel the meds. Once done, I did the Follistim pen, easy peasy. I didn't have to take the Lupron in the morning, only in the evening. I do have to remember though that it is only 5 units now versus 10 :-o. After my shower, I took my prenatal and the antibiotic. I ate a banana while driving to work. Boy, my stomach started doing all kinds of tricks by the time I got to work. I became extremely nauseous and thought I was going to pass out. It was awful. I had to eat some of the plantain chips I have "in stock" at the office. After about a full hour of discomfort, I started to feel better. So, tomorrow, definitely no antibiotic until after lunchtime. Now I'm just hoping and praying all continues to progress well. Looking forward to my appointment-filled day on Saturday. I'm just ready to start hearing good news after so much sadness and disappointment. God is good! (BTW, my brother walked out of the DMV with his DL after having it taken away for five years. I'm very excited about that and for him.)

Friday — 05.25.2012 — OMG, thank goodness it's Friday. It's been a long week. But for as much as I watch and stare down the calendar, week's end is already here. When I left the office yesterday, I went directly to church as I had a finance council meeting at 6:30 p.m. The meeting went well.

I arrived home a little before 9:00 p.m. Of course, my ever-so-long routine began: I had to shower, make the bed, prep my meds, figure out dinner, mix my applesauce and probiotic, and finally administer the meds. It wasn't bad at all. Thank goodness for the icepack. When I ice the spot for about five minutes, I do not feel the injections going in. Although the Menopur still burns going in, it's not too bad.

After administering the meds, I ate dinner while I watched the Miami Heat Game 6 at Indiana. It was nerve wracking but WE WON!!! So proud of them. I was then able to watch both last week's and this week's episode of "Mary Mary." Then I watched "Don't Be Tardy for the Wedding." I was knocked out after that. While watching my TV shows, I was experiencing a bit of dizziness and slight nausea, but it was bearable.

I woke feeling tired this morning. I think it was mainly because it's Friday and I am always tired on Fridays. This evening I have to pick up the girls (my nieces) and attend the confirmation rehearsal dinner at the church. I look forward to being home at a decent time tonight as I forgot to do the moxa treatment (per acupuncturist) last night. By the time I remembered, I was already comfortable in bed and couldn't fathom getting up to prep everything and last another 25 minutes being up. I was just too tired.

I look forward to my appointment at the doctor's office in the morning. I am hoping my follicles are looking good and they are growing and responding to the stimulation meds. I also have an acupuncture treatment at 10:00 a.m., which I am looking forward to, as well. But of course it doesn't end there. I have to wash my hair so I have an appointment at the salon after acupuncture. Then I plan to hopefully rest at home for a couple hours before the Mass for the girls' confirmation begins at 5:00 p.m.

(Sigh) As much as I know I have to remain positive and not be a downer, I still can help to want to wonder if this will work this time around. My gut tells me yes but you just never know. I am taking things one day at a time and will wait and see how things progress. I just hope and pray tirelessly that everything works out. Until next time.

Tuesday, 05.29.2012 — It's been a very long, busy, and yet relaxing past three days. So, on Saturday, 05.26.2012, I had an appt for E2 and u/s at 8:00 a.m. That went well. I still have seven follies on the right and five follies on the left. The left ovary also has the cyst. The largest on the right measured at 10mm and the largest on the left measured at 8.8mm. My E2 came in at 169. Because the left ovary had such a big follicle, it served as another indication that the cyst is not affecting anything thus far. After that appt, I drove to my next appt with Dr. Lori Beauchamp for acupuncture. It was also a very relaxing appt. I then drove to my hairdresser and arrived at 11:45 a.m. to get my hair washed. All I have to say is that I didn't leave there until a little after 3:30 p.m. I was exhausted. I then had to arrive at the church by 4:30 p.m. for the confirmation mass of the 8th graders. Mass was lovely. It was done by Archbishop Favalora. He did an excellent job. I felt very renewed and at peace after the confirmation Mass. I then called it a night and rested, watched the Game 7 Celtics/76ers playoff game, a little more TV and then went to bed.

Sunday, 05.27.12, was uneventful. Because I attended Mass on Saturday, I did not attend Mass on Sunday morning. I basically stayed in bed for the majority of the day. I got up to eat and shower in the afternoon a little before 4 p.m. I then caught the Game 1 of OKC/Spurs playoff game for the Western Conference Finals. It was a really good game. However, after dominating for most of the game, OKC lost.

I woke up at 6:00 a.m. for my 7:15 a.m. appt on Monday, 05.28.2012. I wasn't too bad in arriving as I got there at 7:20 a.m. My follies look good. There were still seven on the right and five on the left. The biggest on the right came in at 13.4mm and 13.0mm on the left. Also, the cyst got smaller on the left side, YAY, great news!! I called phone tree and my E2 came in at 511! It means things are cooking in there. I figured this to be true as until I empty my bowels, I feel the pain pressure of the expanding ovaries. It's not pleasant, but it's bearable. I'll do anything, so I'm not complaining. I just take each day and symptom and ailment one step at a time. Phone tree indicated that the doctor wants me to keep the same dosage of meds: (PM) Follistim 75 and Menopur and then (AM) Follistim 75 and Menopur 75. I am then to go in at 7:00 a.m. on Monday morning for a repeat E2 and u/s and the pre-op consult with the nurse.

So, I went in this morning and arrived at 7:10 a.m. Ms. Paula drew my blood and Ms. Colleen did the scan. Everything went well. I then waited for the nurse and was called in by Nurse Lucy. She took my vitals and went over the questionnaire so we can update accordingly. She explained that I now have seventeen, YES 17, follicles!! There are nine on one side and eight on another.

I was blown away! On top of that, the biggest ones are already at 16, 15, and 13. So things are really cooking in there, as evidenced by my bloated and slightly sore lower abdomen. Based on my progress, it seems I may have two or three more days of stims before the trigger, then retrieval. I'm getting excited but still trying to keep the raw emotions at bay: one day at a time. I'm currently waiting (11:45 a.m.) for phone tree to be updated with my E2 results and game plan for tonight and when to come back for repeat labs and u/s.

Phone tree was finally updated and I obtained the results from the morning's visit. My E2 came in at 749. There are 19 follicles. Nadia asked for me to call the office to let them know if I want to proceed with PGS. I called and spoke to Nurse Gina. I advised her that because my Counsyl results came back negative, we've decided not to proceed with PGS. I asked if Dr. H. mentioned anything, and she explained that normally if everything comes back OK, then he doesn't make a note and it's basically up to us. I then asked Gina about my lining. She explained that it was 6.7 and the prior scan showed it at 4.8. So things are indeed cooking in there. I asked what was considered good and she said that anything above 7 is good and that I was basically just about there.

Wednesday, 05.30.2012 — I took all my meds as instructed last night and then again this morning. I am really feeling more discomfort in my lower abdomen area. I must also say that I have so much EWCM (egg white cervical mucus) that it's just baffling. I started feeling a bit of moisture and it is from the abundance of CM (cervical mucus) that is being produced. They say it's a good sign, so I'm happy about that.

I called Walgreen's to fill the remainder of the Rx that Dr. Hoffman gave me a few weeks ago. It contained the Medrol, Z pack, and Levaquin. These meds are necessary effective after the retrieval. I hope to pick them up tomorrow afternoon or Friday morning. I have to remember to call in and request to fill the Crinone at Walgreen's Margate. I hope to pick that one up this week or this weekend.

This cycle has been a bit different than the last cycle. Last time, I did not feel any pressure or anything while on the meds. It even made me think that I wasn't responding, but in fact I was. With this cycle, I started to feel the cramping and pressure while on the meds since maybe after five days of stimulations. I actually thought that because I already have a 16 and some 15s, that they'd have me come back today for another scan. They didn't. I'm due to go in tomorrow morning at 7:30 a.m. I think they may agree for me to trigger tomorrow night or Friday night, depending on the E2 levels and the # of follicles that have grown to between 18–21mm. I am hoping that it's in God's will that we have a successful cycle that results in healthy baby(ies) and I'm able to attend my niece's graduation. With that said, I hope and think that I'll trigger Friday night. That'll put my retrieval for Sunday morning and the transfer would strive to be on Friday morning of blastocyst embies. Either way, I will continue to pray that all goes well and just take it from there...OK, until tomorrow.

Thursday, 05.31.2012 — Today is Thursday. Based on the size of my follicles this morning, I do not think I will trigger this evening. I still have nineteen follicles: 11 on the right and eight on the left. The biggest on the right measures at 19.5mm. The biggest on the left measured at above 18mm. I then met with Nurse Nadia. She is really nice. She printed the results from the scan and reviewed them with me. She explained that if we count all the follicles that are currently at 15mm or above, we should have about nine to work with. She was really pleased with my response to the stimulation meds. She says that if my E2 doesn't come in too high today, then the doctor will probably keep me on the meds for one more day.

I asked Nurse Nadia about going for a spa day (Sat, 06.02) that was planned by Maria & Anne for my birthday. She said that she would not recommend doing a massage. She explains that she doesn't want anything to get stimulated and have a possible negative effect on what's going on with my ovaries, blood flow, etc. I am taking their advice and staying put. Thank God Maria was able to call and reschedule the spa day for mid-Oct and include a prenatal massage versus a regular massage ☺. I pray all is successful with this cycle and I have a healthy uneventful pregnancy and bring home healthy babies (deep breath). I am waiting for phone tree to be updated so I can get my E2 levels and further info from the Dr.

Judy called and left message on phone tree. My E2 came in at 2,054! What a huge jump from Tuesday's number. It's a good sign. I called back to ask about my lining and Nurse Bonnie said it was 6.7mm. I told her that seemed to be the same measurement from Tuesday and she agreed it was kind of weird. She called me back after discussing with the Dr and they are not worried. They explained that Tuesday's measurement was a bit more generous (??). We'll just wait and see how tomorrow's lining looks.

My dose for Thurs p.m. was changed. I am to take 5 units of Lupron, 75 IU of Menopur but 0 Follistim. Friday morning I am to take 75 IU of Menopur and 75 IU of Follistim. My appt is for 7:45 a.m. on Friday.

Friday, 06.01.2012 — Thank goodness it's Friday! I am so exhausted and feeling very bloated and achy. I was late to my appt this morning. I barely made it out of the house this morning. I arrived at 8:05 a.m! All went well. Amelia drew my blood. She is very nice and easy to talk to. She's from Boston, so we were talking about the Heat/Celtics series. Then my ultrasound was done and all looked OK. I asked to see the nurse to see what the plan may be for the trigger shot. Nurse Bonnie was very helpful. She printed out the ultrasound report that showed all my follicles that were measured and the lining, which came in at 7.3mm today. She thinks I may trigger tonight or Sat night. She explains that because I have a previous cycle, they may compare the stats to see if they will allow me to go one more day on meds to get more mature follicles.

I asked Nurse Bonnie about having an extra vial of Menopur on hand. She was nice enough to check for me. I have 225 IU of Follistim remaining. However, I have only one more Menopur remaining. I can use it tonight if I don't trigger. I would have been short one Menopur for the morning dose. I was very thankful she was able to find one. She did say that if I did not need to use it to please bring it back to replenish the "donor" stock. I happily agreed☺.

Bonnie also said that if I am going to trigger tonight, the nurse (Debbie) would call and speak with me. She says they normally also leave a message on phone tree but they also like to speak directly to the patient to ensure they get all the instructions correctly. I am now in waiting mode: either to listen to phone tree message or speak with the nurse when she calls. Until later.

Nurse Debbie called a little after 1 p.m. today. My trigger is indeed going to be for tonight. This means that my retrieval is scheduled for Sunday morning. My DH and I have to arrive at the Margate office at 8:15 a.m. I have to go for a blood draw at 7:15 a.m. tomorrow. They'll be checking to ensure the hCG shot is actually in my system.

Mary Anne Wood (my HR Dir friend) has agreed to give me the trigger shot. It must be given precisely at 10:30 p.m. tonight. DH had to ensure he was all clear as well so things can be nice and fresh for Sunday. Of course, I call to tell him this after speaking with the nurse and when I called him back about three hours later, he had still not taken care of it. I was furious. He then figured as much because he hung up and then tried to call me back and make small talk. I'll just speak with him later when I leave the office. These men only have ONE thing to do for this entire process and they can't even do that!!! It's very frustrating. But he'll definitely get an earful from me later on.

The nurse said that I did not have to take any meds tonight at all as it relates to the Lupron, Menopur and Follistim. YAY!!! Nothing to eat or drink after midnight Saturday night. Sunday morning, I am to take my Levaquin with a little sip of water on my way to the clinic. I have acupuncture scheduled for 2:30 p.m. tomorrow with Dr. Eubank. I am really looking forward to it as I'll be very relaxed and a bit more ready for Sunday. I'm just continuing to hope and pray that everything goes well and this results in a successful cycle. It's all in GOD's hands.

Saturday, 06.02.2012 — My appointment was at 7:15 a.m. at the Margate office. They are going to check my E2 level and hCG level. Nurse Erica left the message on phone tree for me. My hCG was 152 and my E2 was 3,521. So, Mary Anne and I did a great job administering the hCG injection last night. I must say I was EXHAUSTED. I'm not even sure how I woke up and made it to the clinic. I got home a little before 9:00 a.m. I tried to stay up and watch TV, why, I don't know, but my body couldn't take it anymore. I was knocked out and did not wake up again until 1:30 p.m. I then got ready for my acupuncture appt at 2:30 p.m. My hubby drove me there. The rest of the day was pretty uneventful. We ran some errands and I was home early and went to bed. I must say that my husband went out and he got home a little after 4:00 a.m. So we started talking and he was asking if I was nervous about the next day. I wasn't until he started talking about it. I was ready. I started feeling that because I couldn't feel the pain/pressure in my ovaries that I ovulated early. I immediately took those thoughts out of my mind because I figured even if I did; I couldn't do anything about it anyway. Needless to say, I didn't really sleep much after that.

Sunday, 06.03.2012 — We drove to the clinic and checked in at the second floor. Nurse Judy was there and explained she remembered us from last year. My husband immediately remembered her, but I didn't. She asked about how the last cycle went. I explained to her that we did, in fact, get pregnant. She asked about the baby. I then explained that we unfortunately lost the baby at 22 weeks. She was very empathetic toward us. I told her the whole story. She then explained that she had two losses as well but hers were early on and she did not have infertility issues so she can't even imagine what we went through. She proceeded to administer my IV (painless, thank God) and then the anesthesiologist came by to speak with us.

I was first up that day. Dr. VW performed the retrieval. It was nice that Dr. Hoffman's Medical Assistant, Amalia, was there too, another familiar face. She's really sweet to my husband and me☺. I remember walking into the operating room, being asked to position myself on the bed, confirm/verify my identity, etc. Then I remember Dr. VW telling me I was going to feel the speculum. Then everyone in the room listened in while she asked which is worse, the anesthesia or the speculum. I replied, the speculum. I then remember them debating on how to pronounce my last name. I then told them, "It's easy, think of Duracell battery, but instead of saying 'ell' say 'oh.'" They all laughed and was like, "OK, well that's easy to remember." I don't remember anything else until I woke up next to my husband in recovery.

I don't remember having lots of pain afterward. As the time progressed, however, Judy came to check in on me and asked about the pain, and I said it was like a 6–7. So she gave me two extra strength Tylenol. They told me they retrieved 20 eggs! Yes, 20. So thank God I didn't waste time and energy worrying and stressing about early ovulation☺. I then drank fluids and used the restroom. After I felt a little better, I got dressed. I was then taken downstairs in a wheelchair and we drove home. I had lots of pain after that. It was bearable but it hurt. It was to the point that I started feeling nauseous and began sweating while trying to use the restroom. The nurses forgot to give me the Percocet and Valium Rx. I thought I had some at home from after my delivery but I didn't fill that Rx either. So thank God I had some Tylenol PM and I took two of those. It helped with the pain and I was then also able to get another 3 to 4 hrs. of sleep.

Monday, 06.04.2012 — I am feeling much better this morning. I received a phone call from Nurse Debbie. She explained that of the 20 eggs retrieved, 13 were mature and fertilized with ICSI [intracytoplasmic sperm injection]. Of the 13, six fertilized normally. I was shocked. Debbie explained it was a great thing, but I couldn't help but think I failed somehow. She explained that in order to do a Day 5 I had to have at least three embryos at the 7–8 cell stage with good grading. How do you go from 20 to 6? That's one less than the seven we had last year. She explained that I should check phone tree later in the day for my Day 3 transfer time. She also explained she'd call me on Tuesday between 2 and 3 p.m. to tell me if we're going to go for a Day 5 transfer or stay with a Day 3 transfer. In the meantime, I emailed Nurse Erica and she called me back by 4ish. She said that everything looked good and to not be discouraged at the #s. She explained that is why they aim for 15–20 eggs so that they can aim toward a # of eights being mature and get 50% fertilization from there, so I was in a good place, according to their criteria and goals. Speaking with her made me feel better.

Tuesday, 06.05.2012 — I am anxiously waiting the call from Nurse Debbie. She called in the afternoon and said that the lab was not able to determine yet if I'll go Day 3 or Day 5. She said that I have four that are right on track and the other two are still alive but are a little behind. She asked me to be ready by 8:30 a.m. when she called. That way, if the lab wants me to come in then I'll be ready and not delay the process. So needless to say, I felt again helpless and just prayed every minute asking God to do what he felt best to get us a positive result. In the meantime, I had a 6:30 p.m. acupuncture appointment with Dr. B. She was really sweet and took her time to listen to my drama and helped me feel better as well. The treatment went well too. I didn't leave there until 8 p.m. I went home feeling much more relaxed and being happy that I had the pre-retrieval appointment, just in case.

Wednesday, 06.06.2012 — Ok, so as much as I felt in my gut that I'd have a Day 5 transfer, I was also ready for the information and instructions I was going to hear on the other end of the line when Nurse Debbie called. She called at 8:24 a.m. I was already dressed and ready. She explained that the lab said the transfer will be done TODAY. She explained that of the four that were on target yesterday, only two of them reached the 7–8 cell criteria, not three. So because of that, they want to put back those two ASAP.

I woke my husband up and told him it's time to go. He got ready and we headed out. I stopped at Publix and purchased my whole pineapple. We drove to Margate and stopped at the Walgreen's first so I could pick up the Valium Rx that Debbie called in for me on Monday when I told her the nurses forgot to give me the Rx. After that, we drove across the lot to the clinic. We arrived at the second floor and checked in.

I had to drink four more cups of water on top of the ¾ bottle I had to drink on my way there. They had us sign consents for cryopreservation papers, etc. They then provided us with a picture of the two embryos. The grading scale: 1st # is how many cells, 2nd # is grade from 1 through 6, one being excellent. Mine were graded 82 and 72. She said that the 7 cell was probably most likely already an 8 cell since they checked them earlier in the morning. She explained that they are perfect! I was very happy to hear that. I then took the Valium and started to feel a little woozy. My wanted to empty my bladder a little bit but the Dr. was ready for me so it was time for to go. I walked in to the operating room at about 11:20 a.m. or so (just estimating). The entire team was there. I was happy to see what it was Dr. Barrionuevo that was doing the transfer, as he was the one to do it last time. He was very empathetic after reading my chart. He said we'll do our best again for a positive result. He said unfortunately there is no way to know about these issues until they happen so now everyone will be more aware and cautious regarding my pregnancy. They asked about my o/b. I told them I saw Dr. Martin, and Dr. Hoffman recommended Dr. Salih Yasin from University of Miami's Jackson Memorial Hospital (UM/JMH). He and the other residents in the IVF O/R said that's why they were asking about my O/B because they'd recommend Dr. Yasin as well. They said feel good that Yasin is the one that trained Martin and who is training all of them. Dr. Barrionuevo then talked us through the transfer and he said my endometrium (lining) looked perfect. I was able to see what he was doing on the ultrasound screen. He then explained, OK, we've done what we can and now you know it's no longer up to us but up to the Big Guy upstairs. Men of science who put GOD first is just extremely telling of the kind of practice these doctors are running. That made us feel good. I was then transferred from the o/r bed to my recovery bed and lay there, with the foot of the bed higher than the head of the bed, for 30 minutes. I really had to use the restroom but I definitely waited a little past my 30 min.... I then used the restroom and inserted my Crinone. I then got dressed and we left. I got home and rested the entire day. I got up to use the restroom and to eat dinner for about 15 minutes or so. And now, I just pray profusely, morning, noon, and night.

Friday, 06.08.2012 — I had an 8:00 a.m. appointment this morning to check my P4 (progesterone) levels. Amalia drew my blood and recommended I speak with the IVF Nurse regarding what levels I need to have that are considered good. I spoke with the nurse and she said anything above 5 was good since I was using the Crinone. I then drove home, made breakfast, and became a couch potato. I checked phone tree around noon time and Nurse Nadia left me a message. She said that my levels came back at above 40! She said they like to see above 10, and I was definitely doing great. She said all looked well and to keep doing what I'm doing and wished me luck at my pregnancy test appt. I was elated to hear that because I just didn't know what to expect. It just sounds like my body is also producing the hormone correctly in addition to the Crinone I am using. Thank you, God. I pretty much rested the remaining of the day.

Saturday, 06.09.2012 — Saturday morning is here. My husband and I basically lay around the house all day and did nothing. He took my car to the car wash and came home and took another nap. We woke up around 7 p.m. to get ready to go to our friends Julie and Damien's home to watch the Game 7 match-up between the Miami Heat and the Boston Celtics. I haven't seen my friends in over three months, and I don't really get out of the house so it was good to be out there. The evening went well. The Miami Heat, our team, WON! I promised to not overexert myself and use too much energy as I wanted to remain stress free☺. We got home at about midnight. My husband went out to meet with his dad at a birthday party and I stayed home, watched TV, and then fell asleep.

<u>Sunday, 06.10.2012</u> — I was up a little before my 9:00 a.m. alarm. I then got ready and dressed for church. My hubby ditched me as I think he got home really late and was unable to wake up to go to Mass. My nieces and nephew were able to go, so I was able to sit with them. The Mass was great, as usual. I then drove to my in-laws' home and stayed there until Sunday dinner was ready. My hubby showed up around 1:00 or so, if I remember correctly. I started having some cramping, but it was bearable. I didn't have any cramps last time. So I wasn't sure what to make of them. We left there a little before 5:00 p.m. I then got home, changed, and got in bed. I must have been tired because I feel asleep a little after 5:00 p.m. and didn't wake up until 9:40 p.m. (due to my phone ringing). My cramps were pretty much gone by the time I woke up. I then started prepping for the work week while watching all of my Sunday night show line-up. My husband then came home, and we watched a little more TV and talked. I realized it was 2:00 a.m. when I started to watch "The Client List" on Lifetime. So, I just turned off the TV and tried to sleep. I tossed and turned for a while until I finally fell asleep.

Monday, 06.11.2012 — Again I was up much before my 8:00 a.m. alarm. I was up at 7:19 a.m. I just started my morning routine of getting ready for work. I arrived at my office at 8:35 a.m. I had this overwhelming feeling of not wanting to be there. So, I made the coffee and basically retreated to my office and closed my door. I am feeling a little better now as I am ready to go home. Although, I am trying to focus on work and trying to get things done since I was out three days last week.

A little before 1:00 p.m., I called the clinic and spoke to Nurse Debbie. She told me the report I got on Sat of the one frozen blast was basically the final report. She said it was great as only about one in three patients ever gets any embryos to freeze. I asked her about the grade of the embryos and she explained that they didn't indicate the grade in the computer. She says that for them to be frozen they have to be graded between 2 and 5 and be As and Bs. She said that when it's time to thaw them, I'll be able to get a grade. She said that's because is traumatic to them to be frozen and then traumatic again to thaw. So after they thaw, they let them expand for 4 hrs. and then assign a grade.

I am feeling OK now. Not having many symptoms at all. It's just hard to read into any symptom or lack thereof because you just never know. I am just trying to remain positive and faithful that my babies are responding well to my body, which should do what it is here to do.

I asked Nurse Debbie about the Beta testing being only nine days post my transfer as I was a little concerned that it was too early. My last cycle was a Day 5 transfer and my beta was 10 days later. She said that the dates are carefully calculated, and I should not worry about it as they determine the beta test date based on the date of the hCG trigger injection.

I also asked if I could pay the $1,500 cryopreservation fee when I'm at the office on Friday. She said I can pay then or if I wanted to pay earlier I can contact Joy, the billing manager, at (954) 247-6208, and pay via phone. I spoke with my husband, and we're going to pay on Friday when I'm at the office...Until tmrw....

Tuesday, 06.12.2012 — Ok, so I made it another day. This whole waiting thing is so very difficult to do. I'm still not sure how I made it through last cycle, now that I think about it. Thank goodness the days are going by well and quickly. Although, sometimes I wish they'd go by even faster but it's OK☺. I am not really feeling any noticeable symptoms. Last night I felt a bit of fullness in my lower belly area. When I woke up this morning, I had a bubbly belly as well but no cramping or anything. I felt some slight twinges this morning but nothing else out of the ordinary. I say this because I really don't want to get into analyzing symptoms or lack thereof because if you do that, your mind will really start playing tricks on you. So, it all goes back to the fact that you just have to wait until testing day.

I had, what I think, was implantation bleeding/spotting last cycle. It occurred on 5dp5dt and on 6dp5dt. If I follow the same timeframe with this cycle and indeed have implantation bleeding/spotting, it will be on 7dp3dt and 8dp3dt, which will be on Wed, 06.13.12, and Thurs, 06.14.12. I must remember, too, that not everyone has implantation bleeding and not every cycle is alike, so I'm trying not to read too much into having it or not having it either. (Sigh)

I emailed my acupuncturist Dr. Duro and she had some really inspiring and positive words to help motivate me today:

> Hi Marline,
>
> Congrats on the frozen embryo! That means it was very good quality, as they usually will not freeze it otherwise. I know this is the toughest time—the waiting game—but hang in there and do your meditations during acupuncture and while at home if possible. I will keep you in my prayers and look forward to seeing you this weekend.
>
> Remember, your body knows what to do. Trust that it is healthy and that all will go as planned :-) all the best,
>
> Dr. F Duro

After reading this, I started smiling from ear to ear. It was very nice to read her message. I am about to have lunch in a little bit and am looking forward to eating once my co-worker returns from Publix. Until tmrw, unless something comes up later on today….

Wednesday, 06.13.2012 — Yesterday was a long day. I was up before my alarm that was supposed to go off at 7:15 a.m.…I got ready and left my home a little before 8 p.m. for my therapy session. I got to work a few minutes after 9:00 a.m. and worked until a few minutes after 6:00 p.m. I then had to gas up my car and run to Ross to look into something for my friend's wedding. Once I left Ross, I drove out west to my acupuncture appointment with Dr. Beauchamp at 7:00 p.m. Acupuncture went really well. Dr. Beauchamp, as well as Dr. Eubank and Dr. Duro, are really positive people. She did a prenatal treatment that was also supposed to help protect my womb like a girdle based on the points she put in. I just know that I felt great afterward and had a little more energy although being tired from a long day. I then had to stop by my friend's house to pick up a gift she wants me to give to a co-worker of mine. I didn't leave her home until after 9:00 p.m. as we were catching up after not seeing each other since the beginning of the year☺. I didn't get home until about 9:30 p.m. I then took my shower, ate a light supper, and got into bed.

Today I am feeling OK. I was experiencing some sharp shooting pains/twinges really low down in my pubic bone/upper vaginal area. I had maybe four or five of those and it hasn't come back since. I'm not sure what that's about. I have to now get through today and tomorrow so I can get to Friday, which is decision day. I feel confident one moment and less confident and defeated the next. This is such an emotional roller coaster. Will continue to try and stay busy at work to get through the work day today and tomorrow. I'm also keeping everything crossed and praying like a mad woman for a positive outcome. I'll add another update later if anything new comes up....

It's about 10:30 a.m. and I now feel like I may be coming down with a cold or something☹. Everyone in the office has been sick and I've thankfully been able to keep it at bay for the past couple of weeks while it went from person to person. I forgot to take vitamin C this morning before leaving the house. Thank goodness that one of the co-workers had some. I hope I don't get too sick as to not negatively affect anything and start feeling better soon.

After taking the two vitamin C tablets, I started to feel a lot better. I must mention though that as the day progressed, the sharp shooting pains in my pubic bone and lower uterine area picked back up again. It was so bad at one point that it kind of took my breath away. They did not last long, but I definitely felt them. Also, when I used the restroom in the late afternoon, I felt pressure and sore(ness) discomfort down there...very weird.

Thursday, 06.14.2012 — It's already Thursday. I thank God for allowing me to make it up to today. That means just one more day until the big day. I am very nervous but am trying to remain calm and positive and letting all things go to God as He and the embies are who are in control now. There is nothing I can do anymore except pray and remain positive and faithful. I am feeling a little weird this morning. I took my prenatal before leaving the house and hadn't had breakfast. But I got really nauseous and my belly was a little upset on my way to work. When I arrived at my office, I had my daily serving of almonds and had two peanut butter cookies/crackers. I am starting to feel a little better now. Not much else to report right now. Just happy today is Thursday, and I am off tomorrow. I'm just hoping and praying everything works out, and we get a positive this cycle.

Forgot to add that upon reading some online posts last night, I found out that one early symptom is an increased basal body temperature. The article explained that when women ovulate, their temperature rises until they start their menses. It remains elevated if a pregnancy is there. So, of course, I checked my BBT last night and it was 98.6 (normal). Then I thought about it, that my body didn't have a normal LH surge for ovulation. My ovulation was forced since I did IVF. On another note though, the morning of my transfer, the nurse checked my temperature and it was 98.3. That was a bit lower than normal. So, I'm not sure if my 98.6 last night could count as slightly elevated. So, I checked it this morning. The basal body temp is checked each morning before you get out of bed and start your day. So, I grabbed the thermometer and while I sat to urinate, I put it under my arms and it came back at 98.8/9. I then just put it in my mouth under my tongue and it came in at 99.1 immediately. So, I'm not sure what that means but figured I'd give it a try...Until next time....

Friday — 06.15.2012 (3wk 5d) — Well, I was up early again this morning. I made it to my appt at 8:01 a.m. Paula drew my blood and verified my cell phone # for the infamous call back. She was very positive and just reminded me that it worked the first time so it'll work again. That made me feel very good, although I was still cautious. I drove to Dunkin Donuts and purchased breakfast. I then went to the Coral Springs mall to shop for my friend's bridal shower gift and an outfit for me to wear to the bridal shower. I had a good time because I got there a little before 9:00 a.m. The department stores were open, but the other stores hadn't opened yet. That worked out fine, too, because I decided to walk around Macy's while I waited for a particular store to open. I'm glad I did because I found a nice outfit and shoes. Everything was on sale! It was wonderful.

I then drove home and began my dreaded wait. I got home by 11:00/11:30 a.m. I can't really remember. Needless to say I was nervous because last year I got "the call" by 11:00 a.m. but it was already after 1:00 p.m. and nothing. Finally, the phone rang at 1:43 p.m. and it was my doctor. He just blurted it out: "Marline, you're pregnant!" It was the best thing I've heard in a long time. I couldn't believe it but was extremely excited. I screamed for my husband to join me in the room (he took the day off to be with me). Dr. Hoffman said my hCG was 219 and progesterone was still over 40! We were extremely excited. I then started to cry from also now being scared, cautious, and anxious at the same time. But I have to trust and have faith that God has blessed us again. I feel good that everything will work out. I'm going to just take things one day at a time and try to see myself at the finish line this time. That's something I didn't do last time. God is great☺. There is just no other explanation for it. I am extremely thankful and will continue to pray.

Monday — 06.18.2012 (4wk 1d) — It's Monday! I haven't been happy about a Monday in a long time. The weekend was good as well. I had a 7:30 a.m. appt at the Dr.'s office. Of course, I was late and didn't arrive until about 7:50 a.m. All went well. I paid the $2K fee for the extended culture for embryos remaining after the Day 3 transfer ($500) and for the cryopreservation of the one that was frozen ($1,500). I then had my blood drawn and she also verified my phone # for the update phone call for later.

I am now at work. I am just anxiously awaiting the phone call to make sure everything looks good. Thank you, God, for everything thus far, and I'm praying for continued positive results.

Something weird happened with my phone. Dr. Hoffman's office finally called at about 1:30 p.m. When I answered the line, I got the recorded message one normally gets when you call the main # instead of actually speaking to whoever was calling. I then immediately got a voicemail message. It was Nurse Erica who called. She told me there was good news and to call back for my blood levels. When I tried to call back, another call from Dr. H's office came in and it was Debbie. She told me that my level was at 1,015! That is so very high. I was expecting it to be around 400–500 because the first one was 219. I hope it means all is still OK. The nurses and doc didn't seem concerned at all and felt the level was great. Either Debbie or Erica scheduled me for my next hCG level on Thursday, 06.21.2012, at 7:45 a.m. Debbie explained it would be my last beta. She also explained that I need to schedule the first ultrasound for the following week (next week) on either

Tues, 06.26, or Wed, 06.27. I was able to get an appt for Wed, 06.27.2012, at 10:00 a.m. If my estimates are correct, I'd be five weeks and three days then. I thought it was a bit early, but I think they want to confirm the pregnancy and hopefully be able to see if there is only one little baby or two☺. I am continuing to pray that the next set of levels come back OK on Thursday. Then I just have to get through the weekend so we can go to the ultrasound appt.

As far as symptoms go, I really don't have much. I feel my heart rate a lot and it seems a bit elevated. I'm a little tired but I'm not falling asleep at my desk yet, LOL. I have some pain/discomfort in my ovaries/uterine area. Also, if you were to look at my belly it seems a bit swollen and I think it's because so much is going on in there and I'm not totally back to normal after the retrieval. Last cycle, the swelling, etc., went away by the time I was about 6/7 wks along. Also, I have a bit of increased cervical mucus when I wipe, but it looks like the remnants of the Crinone gel that I have to insert vaginally each morning. It likes to work its way out as the day progresses.

I'll be leaving my office in about 15 minutes and am looking forward to resting a little early this evening.

Tuesday, 06.19.2012 (4wk 2d) — There is not really much to report today. I was up early and arrived at the office a little after 8:30 a.m. The day was pretty much uneventful. I had fruit and nuts as a breakfast snack: totally delicious. After eating that, I was doing my countdown to lunchtime. After work, I had an acupuncture appt. The treatment was really good, as usual. I must say though that I became a bit emotional when Dr. Beauchamp asked how I was doing and how I was taking everything in thus far. I started thinking about Baby Angel Grace. She was very comforting and explained that how I was feeling was normal because I'll never ever forget her. She then also recommended a book called *Heaven Is for Real*. She said it talked about a little boy who was fighting a serious illness and happened to go to heaven and was blessed to come back to the real world. She said that when the little boy came back, he was telling his mom about Jesus, what heaven looked like, and that he saw his sister. The mom was in shock because she said she had never told him (as he wasn't old enough to know anyway) that she had a miscarriage before having him. Dr. Beauchamp really reinforced the fact that Baby Angel is still here with me in spirit and she indeed lives on. She really wanted me to read the book as she thought it'd give me inspiration and help me to feel better.

After leaving my appt, I had to stop by my in-laws' to take care of some online bill pay. I didn't take my normal route home. The route I took just happened to be part of the route I took on my way home from the hospital after I had Angel. The flood gates just popped open. I could not contain my emotions and tears. All of the thoughts and memories of the entire tragic event just came back to me all at once and was as clear as day☹. It was as if I was reliving the entire situation again.

I finally made it home after grabbing some supper/dinner. I didn't even want to really talk to my husband either. Although taken aback, as he hates when I am sad, he gave me my space and didn't call. After showering and taking care of some quick chores, I was in my bed. I felt much better after that. I just prayed for God to continue to be with us while we go through this.

Wednesday, 06.20.2012 (4wk 3d) — It's Wednesday. This means I have one more day until my next beta hCG level blood test. I just pray that all turns out to be OK. I am actually feeling pretty good. I have no real pregnancy ailments, per se. I have to note that when I went to the restroom late morning, there was nothing on my liner, which is great. However, when I wiped, there was light pinkish/red. I kind of freaked out but figured I'd just watch it to see how it progressed and prayed it just stopped. I tried calling the nurses but they were having a meeting and thus I was unable to speak with anyone. In the meantime, I had lunch. After lunch, I went to the restroom and still nothing on the liner, thank God. When I wiped, the spotting was significantly lighter and much less. I cleaned myself up a bit and am just determined to remain positive and pray it just goes away all together.

The reason why I get freaked out with any bleeding/spotting is because of my previous experience. Although everything turned out OK, there was so much blood that each time I just thought "OK, that's it, I'm no longer pregnant." I happened to ask my sis-in-law today, who's pregnant, if she experienced spotting. She doesn't know I'm pregnant. Also, she got pregnant the natural way. She said that she experienced no spotting/bleeding at all thus far (She's about 22wks along). I then tried to rationalize the fact that IVF patients probably have a tendency to have more incidences of spotting/bleeding due to the progesterone suppositories. Since my uterus is growing and the baby(ies) is/are burrowing in even more, then that may be what's causing some light pink spotting to present itself. I'll ask the nurses about my theory when I speak with them.

I have my next therapy session later today at 4:45 p.m. I can't wait to talk to Dr. Gotthelf. After that, I am visiting someone in the hospital. She had a procedure called "the Sleeve." It's along the lines of a gastric bypass/lap band used to aid in weight loss. After that I am off to my home where I'll just lie down and relax until tomorrow morning.

Therapy was great. My therapist was on pins and needles waiting to find out the results. She said she'd try to call me back but was experiencing some difficulties with the phone. I told her she probably was calling a bad number because the office managers were able to contact me just fine to confirm my appointment. When I told her the news, she was extremely excited and happy for me. She told me she thought about me the entire weekend as she realized it was Father's Day. She said she thought, "Oh my, since Mother's Day was such a horror and torture for Marline, I hope that Father's Day is a good one." She was right. It was a wonderful Father's Day. After speaking for a little while, she decided to do a relaxation treatment to help me with the anxiety and stress. She attached the probes to my head and fingers and we began the treatment. It was very relaxing. The results were also favorable in that my stress level from beginning to end flat-lined. It was a great experience.

Thursday, 06.21.2012 (4wk4d) — I was up at 6:30 a.m. this morning. I made it to my appt on time, which was great. Ms. Paula drew my blood and expressed how happy she was for me☺. Then I checked out and was on my way to work. I arrived at the office by 8:42 a.m. I then sat at my desk contemplating how I'm going to make it through until the afternoon to find out my results. A little before 10:30 a.m., my phone rang and it was Dr. H's office. Nurse Debbie told me my levels came in at 2,343. I asked if that was good for how far along I am and she said it was a good level. I compared my results to last year and at 4 weeks 6 days my levels were 1,740. I am four weeks four days today and the levels are 2,343. I think that is a good sign. I have taken a huge sigh of relief, at least for now. I am constantly thinking and hoping everything is OK. I'm glad to know that God is working with me and allowing me to see that all will be fine and will continually be fine.

I am still feeling fine. My breasts are full but not sore. I still have no nausea/morning sickness (just like last pregnancy, thank God). I am feeling some pulls, twinges, crampy/aches at times but nothing prominent or serious. I just get extremely hungry if I haven't eaten. I'm also glad to report that after using the restroom a little while ago, there was no pink spotting/bleeding☺. I just pray that it continues to stay away.

I started to feel a little restless as the day went on. My coccyx bone is really starting to ache from the fact that I sit for 8–9 hrs a day at my desk. I have researched online to find a support pillow I can utilize to help alleviate the discomfort.

I've been counting down the hrs/mins until I can go home. I feel so tired and ready for my bed. Today was also one of those weird days in that it marked exactly six months since the delivery of my baby girl Angel Grace. I miss her so much and think about her daily. I often wonder how my life would be now if she were here. What would she be like personality-wise? Would she still look like her father? Would she still have some of my features? I must say though that God works in mysterious ways, and thus we are very happy right now to have been blessed again with another miracle of life. I just try to remain positive and continue to pray that all goes well with this pregnancy. This has indeed been a very crazy, traumatic, emotional, heart-wrenching, and difficult time in our lives. I'm going to try and listen to my husband and friend to try not to stress as there is nothing I can do to change things at that particular moment. I try to immediately think positive thoughts and then go in to thanking God for all I have thus far and for what He's doing for us. That makes me feel better instantly.

Friday, 06.22.2012 (4wk5d) — It's Friday!!!!! It is an exciting day in south Florida, especially Miami. The Miami Heat has won the 2012 NBA Championship! I was up until after midnight last night, fighting my sleep the entire time, in order to catch this historical moment. LeBron, Wade, Bosh, Chalmers,

Haslem, Miller, Battier, Howard, Jones, Cole, Anthony, and all of the players, including Pat Riley and Eric Spoelstra, have done a tremendous job this year and made it all the way to the end. I am extremely proud of them and even happier for them that they were able to accomplish this goal and reach their dream of an NBA Championship after so much hate, negative talk, animosity, etc. God is good!

I arrived at my office a few minutes after 8:00 a.m. I'm trying to aim toward leaving by 5:00 p.m. to make it to my 5:30 p.m. acupuncture appointment. I feel pretty good and have no ailments thus far. Thank God for that! I must say I am looking forward to lunch time in order to chow down☺.

Monday, 06.25.2012 (5wk1d) — OK, so it's Monday, which means I made it through the weekend. The weekend was pretty good. After acupuncture on Friday, I came straight home. I took a shower and I think I got in bed because I was so tired and called it a week. I was up at 6:16 a.m. on Saturday morning. There wasn't much to watch on TV that early but I made it through. I wanted to go to the grocery store but it rained the entire morning. A little after 2 p.m. I went across the street to my hairdresser in order to wash my hair. I got home at about 5:30 p.m. We stopped at my in-laws' house for about an hour. We then went to the grocery store. After that we got home and got ready for dinner with a few friends. By the time we got home it was after midnight.

Sunday was good, but it was also a long day. We woke up in time to make it to 10:00 a.m. Mass. Then came home and did a little laundry and watched movies. We then went to my in-laws' to have dinner around 3:00 p.m. After that we went to visit my husband's best friend's mom who had a leg amputation. When we returned home it was about 7:00 p.m. I finished up laundry for that day, ate supper, and got into bed. I was really tired. Plus, my coccyx bone was acting up.

Today I am feeling fine, thank God. I have just one more work day to get through until my first ultrasound with Dr. Hoffman on Wednesday. This evening I will cook for the first time in a long time. I also made a dental appt. After discussing it with Mary Anne, she strongly suggested I speak with the Dr. before attending the appt. She explained something about bacteria being released from the gums during the cleaning that may not be good for the baby if it's swallowed. On the flip side, I read a week 5 pregnancy article and it explained that this week one should schedule a dental appt and be sure to tell them you're expecting. So I'll just wait until Wednesday to confirm with Dr. Hoffman on how to proceed.

As far as symptoms go, nothing really to report. My breasts are very full and heavy but not really sore. Nipples are more pronounced and areola is very dark. No nausea, vomiting, spitting, etc. I'm just a bit more tired and that's all. Really hoping it stays that way, just like last pregnancy, but also hoping all is still going well inside there and the little one(s) are holding on and developing as they should. I forgot to mention that the weird dreams are back. When I was pregnant the first time, I kept having the weirdest dreams. Some of them were scary, funny, totally bizarre, etc. They were just all over the place. This time is no exception. Last night I dreamt we were having triplets! Yes, triplets! I saw it as bright as daylight in the dream on an ultrasound monitor. They were playing with each other and just rolling all over the place☺. I'm not sure what that means but hoping again the ultrasound on Wednesday goes well.

Tuesday, 06.27.2012 (5wk2d) — It's Tuesday. I am feeling OK today. I have a very bubbly and gassy belly but totally fine otherwise. I think I may have overdone it last night. I made dinner, did two loads of laundry, cleaned the fridge and washed dishes. By the time I got into the shower and then lay on the sofa to rest, my body had had enough. I was very achy and happy to have been resting by then. There is not much more to report. I was up early again this morning. I was able to make breakfast, wash my one leftover pot from last night, fold last night's load that was in the dryer, and watch a little TV news before getting ready for work. I have acupuncture tonight and am looking forward to that. Tomorrow is the big day. Surprisingly, I am not nervous, yet. I am just trying to think positive and remain faithful that everything will be OK. It's funny because last year this time, I really had no unusual worries at all. I was always a little nervous going into appointments but that was because I was dealing with the unknown. This time around the nerves are a bit more different. So, I'm really just continuing to hope and pray that all goes well.

<u>Wednesday, 06.27.2012 (5wk3d)</u> — So, I finally made it to the one of many more to come, big days. Surprisingly, I was not really nervous. I think my belly felt otherwise as when were we ready to walk out of the house I had to use the restroom. I felt much better afterward. We were about 10 minutes early for our appt. So, we waited after I left a urine sample for the lab to analyze. Analia came to find us and told us that Dr. Hoffman would be with us as soon as he finished up with another couple. In the meantime, she prepped the ultrasound room and then called us in. She held us in nice conversation while we waited. So, Dr. Hoffman then came in and greeted us☺. It's always great seeing him. We then begin the ultrasound and then everyone in the room went quiet, and their eyes/facial expressions started looking weird. So I said, "Ok, I guess something's up since everyone is quiet." Dr. Hoffman then said, "There are two sacs!" I was so shocked, happy, afraid, overwhelmed, excited, etc. All of the emotions were rolled up into one.

Everyone started smiling and laughing and carrying on. Oh, and my first words were "WHAT?!?" Dr. Hoffman continued on with his scan by obtaining other measurements. He said both ovaries were 5cm so still a bit large. I also had free fluid in the abdominal/uterine cavity. He said that is due to mild over stimulation (OHSS). He also said the embryos implanted really high so that's good. I asked about having intercourse and he said not yet until things are a little bit more established. He doesn't want more pressure on the cervix and uterus and from the pushing that goes on as a result. He said I can definitely keep my dental appointment and tell them he said it was OK. He went over the list of items I cannot have while pregnant. Analia then came in with the "packet."

Needless to say, we left the office feeling extremely excited yet scared at the same time. We both agreed that our lives were going to change drastically. But just as God helped us to get here, I know he'll see us through it all the way through.

Dr. Hoffman wants to see me in two weeks. So I scheduled my next appointment for Wed, 07.11.2012, @ 8:45 a.m. He then wanted me to see my OB/MFM, Dr. Yasin @ JMH, in three weeks. I called and scheduled that appointment for Friday, 07.20.2012, @ 10:15 a.m.

Thursday, 06.28.2012 (5wk4d) — OK, so I am extremely tired today. Last night I got this weird pain in my hip/buttock area on the left side and it is still bothering me☹. I called my acupuncturist and she provided some stretching exercises that can help until I see her tomorrow. I did it and it felt a bit better. She said if it wasn't bearable to definitely call so they can squeeze me in tonight. Other than those two ailments, I do not have much more to report for today. I had plans to make dinner tonight but decided against it as I just want to get home and go to bed.

So, I decided to muster up some energy and make dinner. I'm glad I did. It took only an hr. to prepare dinner. I made my shrimp pasta and steamed veggies. It was so delicious. I didn't have any for dinner but I am looking forward to having lunch tomorrow.

The rest of the evening was pretty much uneventful. After my shower, I made the bed and just rested. I was probably asleep by a little after 9:00 p.m.

Friday, 06.29.2012 (5wk5d) — OMG, TGIF. I have been waiting so long for Friday to get here. I am just totally exhausted. The pain in my left glute/hip area has gotten better but had not totally gone away. I am looking forward to my acupuncture treatment later in hopes the pain gets significantly better or disappears all together.

There isn't really much more to report. Oh, it was hard for me to eat my breakfast this morning. I literally had to force it down my throat this morning. I did not have the urge to throw up or anything, which was good, but it was a mission. After eating I felt better. Although I had like a little tummy ache, but it didn't last long, maybe just a few minutes or so.

Five o'clock cannot get here fast enough. After acupuncture, I have a 7:30 p.m. appt for my wax. I'm not going to do my bikini at all. I have to definitely do my face (chin/upper neck), my underarms, and my legs. I totally look like the hairy monster right now. Then I think I'll call it a night after spending some time catching up with my friend. (She is going with me to get waxed.)

I don't have much planned for the weekend. On Saturday, my sister-in-law and I are going shopping for maternity clothes for her to wear. I plan to attend church on Sunday. Also, I'm going to try and get some loads of laundry in. I started last week (shaking my head) and just haven't been able to finish. That's about it. Until Monday....

Tuesday, 07.03.2012 (6wk2d) — It's Tuesday. Where do I even begin? My weekend was pretty uneventful until late Sunday. Friday night, my friend Maria and I went to get our waxes done, after my acupuncture treatment. After waxing, we stopped at T.J. Maxx, and Maria shopped for bathing suits and cotton sun dresses for her honeymoon. We had a good time. When done, we stopped at BK and I must say, I think that must have been the slowest BK I've been to ever. The wait was just awful. And because we were on the beach, there were weirdoes walking around and walking through the cars in the drive through trying to get people to put their windows down to talk to them. That surely wasn't going to happen. We then headed to Maria's home and I got in my car and drove home. By the time I got there, I was exhausted.

Thank goodness I did not have any early morning plans for Saturday morning because I do not know how I was going to get up after such a long week. Nonetheless, my sister-in-law, Anne, stopped by to pick me up and we left the house around 12:30 p.m. She, her best friend, and I stopped at three different stores to help her shop for maternity clothes. In between the shopping we had lunch as well. I returned home by 3:30 p.m. I'm glad I wasn't out too long. I was starting to get a little antsy but caught myself as I remembered she doesn't know I am pregnant as well. A little later in the day my husband and I went for dinner and called it a night.

Sunday morning I woke up for church at 10:00 a.m. Although exhausted, I am glad I went. The message was very powerful and inspirational. I also became very emotional because one of the songs sang was "Amazing Grace" and it took me back to the funeral Mass we had for our daughter Angel Grace. It was very hard, but I felt this overwhelming presence there with me so that made me happy in the end. I returned home and basically took a nap for a few hrs. We then had dinner at my in-laws' home. My husband and I then went to the grocery store, and we were back home and basically stayed in. We watched an awards show and after the awards show, it happened.

I went to bed and my husband told me he'd be right back as he was going to take out the trash for collection Monday morning. A little thereafter, maybe 3 minutes went by, and my brother-in-law knocked on my bedroom door and asked me to come outside cause my husband needed me as our dog was hurt really bad. I immediately put something on and ran outside. I stepped outside of my door to find my poor dog, Speedy, basically lying almost lifeless on the porch☹. It was just awful! By this time, my husband was in the truck trying to go to the dog owner's home that did this to our poor dog. That was to no avail. Because it was already almost 1:00 in the morning, everyone was asleep. I called the police, and they were there relatively quickly. Two officers arrived. They were very upset at what happened. One of the officers started crying as it looked so bad. They advised us to call animal control in the morning and to take Speedy in immediately to the hospital. To make a long story short, Speedy didn't make it. The vet did all he could but to no avail. He explained he already suffered too much internal trauma. It was too much to take in, to say the least, just a sad experience☹.

By the time we got home and settled, it was already 2:00 a.m. I didn't really sleep through the night and had to wake up for work in the morning. I felt awful for my husband as he experienced this awful event, and he was extremely close to our dog.

I arrived at my office on Monday and just couldn't even focus. I was very emotional and basically cried the entire day on and off. I'm not sure if the shock of everything that happened affected me, but I started spotting/light bleed and it was enough to get to my liner. Of course I freaked out. I called my Dr.'s office, and they said not to worry as it's normal and to call back if it gets worse or I have back pain and cramps along with a heavy bleed that's like a period. I resolved myself to not worry about it as it just drove me crazy, and I really did not need that right now.

The spotting basically continued but then it subsided toward the end of the work day.

Tuesday rolled around and I still had the spotting but now it was only when I wiped and thus nothing ever made it to the liner. Also, it was dark red/brown in color so that was good too.

There really wasn't anything else to report. I got home a little after 8:00 p.m. as my acupuncture appt wasn't until 7:00 p.m. I took my shower and got into bed as I was very tired. While in bed, I watched a little TV and then had supper, and I was knocked out after that.

Wednesday, 07.04.2012 (6wk3d) — It's the 4th of July! Thank God for the Independence we have in the great country we live in. Many of us decided to come in to work today for about half a day. I don't really have any other plans. My in-laws may have a BBQ today, but I'm not too sure and I actually doubt that they will. Either way, I plan to leave at around 12:30 p.m. or so. When I get home I am going to try and eat something and then get back in my bed.

I used the restroom earlier and found no spotting on my liner. Then when I wiped, there was nothing on the tissue. So, I am very happy for that today. I'm trying to take things one day at a time. My nurses, and all the reading I've been doing, have explained that spotting/bleeding in the first trimester is very common. They also explain it's even more prevalent in twin and multiples pregnancies. I felt a little queasy this morning and couldn't even stomach the idea of eating breakfast. Yet, I had no choice, I had to eat. I am feeling a little better now, thank God.

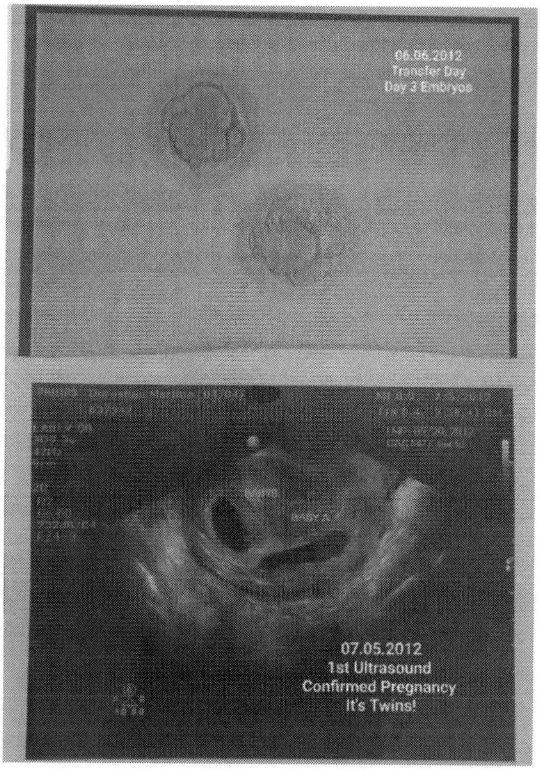

2012, IVF FL Embryology 3-day 7-8 cell embryos for fresh cycle

<u>Tuesday, 07.24.2012 (9wk2d)</u> — Ok, it's been a long time since I've added to this journal. Things have been extremely crazy over the past three weeks or so. The day after 4th of July, I began spotting heavily while at work. I called Dr. Hoffman's office and they asked me to arrive by 2:15 p.m. I had an ultrasound @ 6wk4d and was able to see both heartbeats. It was very reassuring and truly a blessing. I then saw Dr. Barrioneuvo. He said I was bleeding from the opposite side of the lining. I was put on bed rest until Wed, 07.11.2012, which was when my next appt with Dr. Hoffman was. The remainder of the week was pretty uneventful. I had very minimal spotting but followed the orders and took it very easy.

Tuesday, 07.10.2012, rolled around and it was like a faucet had turned on. While lying in bed that morning I felt like I wet my pants. When I stood up, my underwear was soaked. I immediately got into the shower. After showering, I couldn't even dry myself off while trying to get out of the shower as the blood was just streaming down non-stop. It was very light red and I had no pain associated with the bleed. I called Dr. Hoffman's office a couple times but was unable to get through. I just then stayed in bed the entire day. My husband and I figured since we had an appt the next day, we'd just kind of wait and see. I bled for a few more hrs. and then it stopped, and I just had spotting.

The morning of my appt, 07.11.2012, I started bleeding the same way again. I was even unable to give a good urine sample as it was tainted with the blood. Dr. Hoffman did my scan and reviewed the info from my prior week's visit. We were able to see the heartbeats on both babies and they both we measuring right on target, in spite of all the issues I was experiencing. The bleeding subsided and I was still spotting. Dr. Hoffman told me to stay home from work the remainder of the week, and I asked if I could at least work a few hours at my office. He nodded his head and said, "OK." I explained that because I was so tired, I'd take naps at home and it was harder for me to stay up and focus. The remainder of the week was OK. I had spotting every day but nothing crazy. Dr. Hoffman found that I had a subchorionic hematoma and said it needed to work its way out if it didn't get reabsorbed into the lining.

Ugh, that darned subchorionic hematoma again ☹ That is exactly what happened in my first pregnancy with Angel as well. I remember it was just the most scariest experience of my life at the time. It was September 2011. My husband and I were at a wedding where he and his best friend Nervins J were groomsmen in the bridal party. I was about 8 or 9 weeks pregnant at the time. As we waited for the wedding to start, Lourdes (Nervins' fiancé) and I decided to go to the restroom. When I got up from sitting on the 'white' garden chair, I noticed there was a pink stain on it. Embarassingly, I wiped it, as I have sweaty palms – hyperhidrosis – and thus always had a napkin with me. Once in the restroom, my God, it was awful. Quite frankly it was like a bloody scene from hell – like in a horror movie. As I squatted over the toilet and began to use the restroom, I noticed the panty liner I had worn was basically non-existent and soaked. I then heard a large 'bloop' sound of something that fell in the toilet. I was totally panicked at that point. Lourdes is trying to figure out what's going on and how to help. She was unaware I was pregnant. I always knew to not say anything until passing the 1st trimester at least. I let he in the stall with me because at that point I thought I was going to pass out. She was great in helping me get cleaned up. I literally took off my under wear and booties (kind of like boy shorts) and washed them by hand in the sink. I vividly remember Lourdes just being shocked and kept asking "well did you know not your period was going to come?" 😊 I just kept shaking my head in disbelief as I washed up. The great thing is that stall had a hand dryer in it. So after washing my undies, I dried them under the hand drier. Lourdes pointed out my dress was soiled too. It happened that my dress was made of a silk chiffon material. So, I washed that by hand too and stood under the dryer where it dried beautifully. No one could tell I had just cleared up a horror scene. Needless to say, at that point I just know I lost the baby. In my mind, I felt there was no way there could be all that blood and I still be pregnant. I eventually found my husband and told him what happened and he immediately told his best friend and the groom we were leaving. I kept pulling him back to say we could stay because if something did happen, there was nothing we could do anyway. After significant convincing, he reluctantly agreed. I have to tell you the bleeding then just stopped. I was experiencing just a minor trickle and spotting from that moment on.

All in all, we called Dr. Hoffman's office when we got home and they immediately called me back. Because I had no pain, never any pain even with the blood bath, they told me to rest and come in 1st thing Monday. They stressed if anything changed to go to ER and call right away. Thankfully, nothing else really changed. I rested the remainder of Saturday (it was a morning wedding so made it home around 4:30pm) and all of Sunday. When we arrived to the clinic on Monday, as planned, an ultrasound was done and it was ultimately diagnosed as a subchorionic hemorrhage. So yeah, hearing that word again was very triggering for me. I went on to have multiple bleeding spells as the pregnancy progressed but they eventually stopped in the 2nd trimester. I would have weekly acupuncture treatments specifically dedicated to helping stop the abundance of bleeds. I think they helped heal the hematoma faster too. Dr. Duro (Celada at the time) was very tuned in to that treatment for me as well. She definitely helped me through that hectic phase.

So now back to 2012 with the twin pregnancy...

Sunday, 07.15.2012, rolled around. I attended Mass in the morning. Since my husband was still sleeping, I went to my in-laws' house and hung out there. Sunday dinner became ready and I ate. I used the restroom while there and started having a weird spotting. It was mucousy and stringy. I didn't like how it looked, so I went home to get in bed and rest.

I had to put on a pad because I started to have a slight bleed. As the day progressed, it started to get better but wasn't gone all the way. I then attended a baby shower in the early evening. It was the shower for the YANA group founder, Manouchka. While at the shower, I frequently visited the restroom to ensure I was OK. My first trip to the restroom, I was totally having a full-on bleed. After a couple of hours, I was not feeling well, so I left. I got home around 9 p.m. While getting undressed, I sat to use the restroom and that's when my heart just sank. I was wearing an extra-long overnight pad and it was totally soaked with blood☹. I then tried to get up to grab a baby wipe and huge clots fell on my bathroom floor. I didn't know what to do and started to panic. My husband was at work so I was home alone. I cleaned myself up, got in bed, sent a picture of the clots to my husband, said a prayer, and tried to fall asleep. That was no help as I could not sleep. I said I'd wait until my husband came home, and if I was still bleeding we'd go to the ER.

We ended up just calling Dr. Hoffman's office in the morning, 07.16.2012. I still had a full-on bleed. They were able to get me in by 9:15 a.m. Dr. Hoffman checked and both babies were still fine. I was even able to hear heartbeats on both babies. For the first time through this entire bleeding ordeal, I started to cry since morning time while in the shower. I was just sure it was over. How do you lose so much blood and still be OK? But I thank God because he is the only one that got us through this. Dr. Hoffman advised that the bleeding was trying to work its way out and that I may have bleeding for the next two weeks or so and to not panic too much.

He also got back my blood clotting blood work that I had done the week before. Everything came back negative so he/we were all happy about that. I left the office feeling a lot better but definitely not out of the woods yet. He provided me with updated info to provide to Dr. Yasin at JMH.

I saw Dr. Yasin on Friday, 07.20.2012. It was a very good appointment. My husband and I were very happy and felt good about how he was going to watch over our pregnancy.

While at the appointment, Dr. Y checked my cervix with a pelvic exam and saw it was closed. I didn't have lots of blood in there. There was just old blood seeping out that was brownish in color. He swabbed it with a cotton stick and showed it to me. I think he also did a Pap smear. I had a full prenatal panel done with a blood draw and left a urine sample. Overall, the appt went well. He also reviewed my full history and provided some insight and info on how we were going to proceed. He scheduled me for an ultrasound on Wed, 07.25.2012, and a follow-up appt to see him again on Fri, 08.03.2012. That is two weeks from the last appt. He did advise me that I was going to get tired of seeing him. I highly doubt it, as I prefer to be watched closely to ensure all is progressing well, given my history.

Since my last big bleed on 07.15–07.16, I'm happy to say I have not had any more bad episodes. I've just had spotting daily and it's always brownish in color. I just pray that it continues to become less and less and eventually go away soon and that the babies continue to do well. God is great!!

I'm looking forward to my ultrasound appt tomorrow morning. I'm just continuing to pray that all goes well. Taking things one day at a time☺.

<u>Wednesday, 07.25.2012 (9wk3d)</u> — I had my first ultrasound at Dr. Yasin's office this morning. I was a bit nervous but managed to stay calm and remain positive. I was just looking forward to seeing my babies on "TV." The ultrasound went well. The tech was really nice. Unfortunately, I forgot her name. We saw both babies and heard their heartbeats. Baby A was 175 and Baby B was 171. Both babies measured right on target as well. It looks like I still have the bleed. I've actually acquired another one, or maybe she was able to see it for the first time today. She said that for now everything looks good as the babies' heart rates are good. She said you start to worry if the heart rates are low or they are not measuring on target. Thank God they both are doing well. We looked at the cervix. It now measures 4.3cm. It grew from the last measurement of 3.8cm a couple of weeks ago. She told me the cervix was closed but that there was blood hanging in the cervix. She pushed down on my belly a few times and nothing came out on the ultrasound. She said that's good as it confirms the cervix is indeed closed. She explained that the blood is from the bleed and is trying to work its way out. I am very happy. Thank you, Lord God, for all of our blessings thus far and for those to come as well. I now have to try and not worry until my next appt on Fri, 08.03.2012, when I see Dr. Yasin. That date he is going to give us the date for our cerclage to be put in. I'm just praying it's a successful procedure and that all is still well with the babies.

I have not had any bleeding. I am still spotting, but it is still brown and not red. I'm going to continue to watch it until, hopefully, it goes away for good.

Thursday, 07.26.2012 (9wk4d) — It's almost the weekend. Last night was a very busy one for me. I was finally able to get into bed a little before 8 p.m. I started to feel much better when I got to rest a bit. This morning I am still spotting. The spotting was a bit much yesterday after my appt. I think that the probing around via the vaginal ultrasound really got things going in there. The good thing is that it is still brown so still hoping it goes away soon.

I am still spotting today but thus far it's been very minimal. I am started to feel lots of discomfort. I am praying I am able to handle it until my appt with Dr. Yasin next week. My lower abdomen and extremities just ache really badly. I think I am having lots of gas and the discomfort from my coccyx bone is not letting up as I sit without my cushion when I'm not at my office. I am just trying to hang in there and not complain but I spoke with Mary Anne to ask if she experienced this when she was carrying her twins. I now also am having upper back pains. I finally figured out what it must be stemming from. My breasts have grown to double in size and I'm still so early on the in the pregnancy. I find myself slouching a lot and not being able to sit up straight. It's the weight of the heavier breasts that are weighing me down. I will try and purchase sport bras and minimizers to see if that will help a bit.

I got to chat with my hubby when he got home last night/this morning around 3 a.m. We haven't had these talks in a while, so it was nice to talk to him about the babies, our future, finances, etc. Thank goodness I was able to fall asleep again relatively quickly and didn't have too much trouble getting up this morning.

I have a busy day ahead of me today. I have to try and get my eyebrows threaded and then make it to my friend's cousin's home to carpool to the wedding rehearsal this evening. Hopefully I'm not doing too much and can get home by 10 p.m. so I can rest. I'm just continuing to hope and pray to God that all continues to progress well with me and the babies and the pregnancy.

Monday, 07.30.2012 (10wk1d) — I made it through the weekend. It was a very special weekend. One of my best friends, Maria, got married on Saturday☺. It was such a beautiful ceremony and wedding altogether. I was extremely happy and excited for the newly married couple.

I'm starting to feel a lot better as it relates to the colic gas pains I had all of last week. The spotting was also under control during the wedding. I made sure to check every few hours to ensure all was OK. The good thing is that the spotting was still brown in color. I just pray that by the next ultrasound, the subchorionic hemorrhage is totally gone.

Sunday was a great day as well. I woke up in time to make it to church. I took a nap when I got home, and then my husband and I went to get dinner. We then spent some time at my in-laws' and then basically called it a night. I started to get that fullness pain/discomfort in my lower belly. There was also some pain in my pelvic bones too. I also had a bit more spotting in the middle of the night. It kept me up to constantly check to make I was not bleeding. Thank goodness, by morning it had stopped.

I made it in to the office by 10 a.m. this morning. I was also actually able to stay until 5 p.m. I'll be leaving very soon. The spotting has been very minimal today as well, thank God. I'm just hoping and praying it goes away very soon. I am also anxious to see the babies again to make sure they are OK in there. I do say a special prayer for them daily and try to talk to them too, letting them know that God, Mommy, and Daddy love them very much and can't wait to meet them "on time." OK, I'll check back in tomorrow, God willing.

Tuesday, 07.31.2012 (10wk2d) — I'm having a good day today thus far. I must say though, that although I slept from about 6–9 p.m. last night and went back to bed around 1 a.m., I'm still very tired and sleepy. I'm very much looking forward to getting home this evening to get in bed.

The spotting has slowed down significantly. I just hope and pray it continues to stay away altogether. I have also acquired a new symptom. My breasts have been full for a while but they never really hurt before. Lately, the nipples have been extremely sore to the touch. I mistakenly scratched myself last night and I thought I was going to pass out in pain. I have to definitely go for a bra fitting very soon so I can get a bit more comfort. Although, because it's still early, I'm not sure if I'll have to change bras again as I presume the breasts will continue to grow in size. Only time will tell. I'm very anxious but am trying not to worry as I look forward to my next OB appt on Fri, 08.03. I just pray all is well with the babies.

Wednesday, 08.01.2012 (10wk3d) — It's mid-week. Today has been a good day thus far. I've been having some slight discomfort in my lower abdomen area but it doesn't last long and isn't intense. I will definitely mention it to the doc on Fri. The spotting has decreased even further and is very light and brown in color. I'm just hoping it's a great sign that the subchorionic hemorrhage is finally gone.

I must say that the fatigue is getting the best of me. I am sleepy around midday and it returns toward the end of my work shift. I look forward to going home soon so I can get into bed and rest. I've been thinking and wondering about how the babies are doing in there. I will try and continue to be positive and just be optimistic that they are doing fine. I'll be reassured on Fri at my next appointment.

Thursday, 08.02.2012 (10wk4d) — I woke up early this morning and wasn't really tired. I had a very bad dream but glad I woke up to it being only a dream. I just had breakfast and I feel significantly better. As much as I don't feel like eating at times, I have to remember to do so anyway. I started to have the reoccurrence of the colic gas pain this morning but this time instead of being centralized down there, it was more localized to the left side. I definitely want to talk to the doc about it tomorrow.

Although time is flying by, I often feel like I can't wait to hit my next milestone. I really would like to break the news to my sister and my mom. It's just better to wait another week or so just to be further along and at the first trimester mark. God is great and will definitely get us through.

In thinking about delivery, this morning I realized that I may just opt for the C-section, of course if that's what best for us. If I can indeed try to go naturally, my family is going to take it hard but I only want two people in the delivery room. I don't want a repeat of the last delivery where everyone was in my room. At times I didn't care but when it was all over, I felt violated in some ways. It's just weird to have everyone looking into your business. Of course, if my husband can handle it, I'd love him to be there at my head. The other two people would be my sister and original mother-in-law, Nela. (I say original because she is the only mom-in-law I knew, she's my husband's dad's wife, my husband's step-mom before my husband's mom came from Haiti. So now I have 2 mom-in-laws). Everyone else can wait outside until it's all over. I know it's a bit early, but for right now that is the plan.

My cousin Laurie gave me some wonderful advice last night. I have to claim the babies being born and arriving on time. I have to talk to God and continue to thank him for all he's done and get affirmation that this pregnancy will result in healthy and normal babies. I pray that the spotting continues to basically stay away. It's been a few days now and there is not a lot of spotting on my liner at all. We really hope that's the end of it all. Thank you, Lord!

I have my weekly acupuncture treatment tonight and I'm really looking forward to it. It always helps propels me into a relaxed and calm state of mind. Plus, the additional points they do really help with the bleeding. I'm just looking forward to resting as much as I can. It's almost Friday so I'll be back next time, God willing☺.

<u>Tuesday, 08.07.2012 (11wk2d)</u> – So, there are many good things to report since my last update.

My appt with Dr. Yasin was on Friday afternoon. It was a really good appt. Although I did not have an ultrasound, I got to hear both babies' heartbeats. It was such a reassuring, happy, joyous sound. It's just great to know that they are in there doing their thing and growing by the minute. It's truly a blessing, thank God.

Dr. Yasin reviewed my lab results that were taken a week and a half before. All of my numbers and labs came out OK. I was not anemic, which is good, as I worried about all the bleeding I was having. The Pap smear and other vaginal cultures came back negative. We reviewed the ultrasound as well, and he then went on to schedule the date for my cerclage procedure.

He looked at a calendar and chose Wed, 08.15.2012. He chose a Wed so I could be home and in bed the remainder of the week. He said I should be OK to return to work on Monday but that I'll be on restricted pelvic rest nonetheless. He's trying not to confine me to a bed so he wants me to take it very easy and rest as much as I can.

I brought up the subject of delivery and explained I wanted to try and go for a natural vaginal delivery. He explained that for one reason or another, twins are normally delivered via cesarean section 75% of the time. He said it's not to say we cannot try for a natural delivery but there are sometimes risks involved in doing so. He said the only way we'll attempt a natural delivery is if both babies are in perfect position (vertex). He explains that oftentimes, both babies are OK but once the first one is delivered the other one turns which then causes the need to manually turn them or deliver breech, C-section, etc.

He explained that it's still really early, but he's happy I brought it up, although, I need not worry about it too much as we'll ultimately do what's best for both the babies and me. He wants me to focus on more immediate goals like getting through the procedure and going from there.

We talked about a lot of other things that I cannot really remember now but all in all it was another great appointment.

Saturday rolled around and I had all kinds of plans to do chores around the house. Needless to say, that didn't happen. I stayed in bed the entire morning. We left the house to go to IHOP. My mother-in-law cooked for me Saturday morning but by the time I was hungry, I no longer wanted the pasta. We did, however, pick it up on our way home from IHOP. Sunday was also a bit uneventful. I wasn't feeling too hot but made it to church anyway. I'm happy I was able to go to Mass. My nieces and nephew also made it, so that was good, too. When I got home I was able to put in two loads of laundry and that was it. The little kids stayed with me while the two older girls went to the mall. I had the little ones for three hrs. It felt like an eternity as it takes a lot to watch over all of them to ensure they're OK and not getting into any trouble☺. As busy as the baby Ambrielle is, she's so adorable and you can't really be upset with her☺. It was great seeing them. When they all left, I went to bed and didn't get out of bed again until a little after 6:30 p.m.

Monday was also a good day. I must say, though, that work was crazy that day. I was extremely busy from the time I got to work until I left in the evening. The plan was to finish with more laundry, but that surely didn't happen. I took my shower and got on the computer for my in-laws. When they left, I went to bed.

Today, I'm feeling OK, thank God. I'm happy to report that it seems as though the spotting has stopped. I just am sure to watch it and check each time I use the restroom. I think it's a great sign. Let's just hope it stays away for good. I'm taking things one day at a time. God is indeed great!

Wednesday, 08.08.2012 (11wk3d) — Ok, so I started spotting again yesterday evening☹. I noticed it when I used the rest room right before I left for the day. I didn't feel anything so was shocked to see the blood on my liner. It looked old and wasn't a lot at all but to go from having no blood to that, it really freaked me out. I drove home and got there as fast as I could. I took a shower and got into the bed. I consistently checked and there wasn't anything on my liner just a few times when I wiped after using the restroom.

I woke up this morning feeling OK. I still didn't have anything really on my liner but I will continue to check it as the day progresses. I really hope and pray that it's nothing and that the babies are just moving around trying to make more space thus causing the hematoma to now be able to shift its way out. If anything changes, I'll call the doctor's office for reassurance or advice on what to do.

Although I am a bit worried, I am trying to remain positive and not get stressed out. I just hope and pray that God and Angel continue to watch over my babies and keep them safe. I also hope and pray my body holds up and is able to keep them in there until time for them to come home healthy. I have a lot of work to do so hopefully that will keep my mind occupied a bit for the day.

Monday, 08.13.2012 (12wk1d) — I'm feeling a bit nervous today, more nervous than I thought I would be. The rest of last week was pretty uneventful, thank God. I rested basically all day Saturday and did laundry in the evening. Sunday, however, was a very busy day for me. I was up and out all day. I was happy to have gotten back into bed when I did and rested.

I woke up this morning feeling a little nervous about my cerclage procedure scheduled for Wed. I felt the need to tell my mom as I wanted to make sure she knows I was going in for surgery. Plus, I already hit the 12-week mark so I felt a bit better about that too. As of yesterday, I started to have some lower back discomfort. It gets better when I've rested in bed but I cannot stay in bed all day. So, I am going to try and restrict my movements while at work today. I'm looking forward to 5 p.m. so I can go home.

Well I'm going to keep thinking positive thoughts and pray as I know God is with us and will definitely get us through this. I just really want to get the procedure done as I feel it'll provide a little more piece of mind for me knowing that it's in. I also cannot wait until I see the babies on the ultrasound. It's been about two weeks since I saw them, and it just feels like forever. I just hope and pray they are doing well and that my body is holding up its part of the bargain as well. To God be all the Glory!

Tuesday, 08.14.2012 (12wk2d) — Well, I went in for my pre-op appointment this morning. I wasn't sure what to expect but it all went well, nonetheless. The only downside was that my appt was at 10 a.m. and I didn't leave until 10 minutes to 1 p.m.

I met with the financial services department after they received the authorization from the insurance company. I then met with the nurse. She took my vitals. She didn't like my elevated heart rate though. So, she ordered an EKG be performed. Thank goodness that came back "normal." I also had my blood drawn while there.

As nervous as I was yesterday, I am feeling a lot better today. I just cannot wait to see the babies on "TV" tomorrow and to have the procedure done. I just hope and pray it all goes well and that the cerclage actually holds up until the end.

I am feeling tired, so I am happy I'll be leaving my office relatively soon. I was able to break the news to my mom and sister last night. I finally told them we were pregnant and having twins. Both were extremely happy and of course started giving me all the pep talks that I wasn't trying to hear. But they did so because they are worried so I couldn't be mad at that. I feel much better going in to the procedure with them knowing what's going on. When I get home this evening, I'm going to ask my nieces to come over to help me clear up some loose ends around the house before tomorrow.

In the meantime, I've been keeping an eye out on my spotting and it's extremely minimal today. I am very happy about that. It's funny because it's more of a light pink tinged discharge vs. blood. I'm anxious to see what the cervix is measuring tomorrow when I have the ultrasound. Either way, I feel better that it's becoming less.

OK, well I'll be back next week, God willing, with a report of all that took place tomorrow with the procedure.

Thursday, 08.23.2012 (13wk4d) — OK. It's been a little over a week since my last update.

I'm happy to say that my cerclage procedure, performed on 08.15.12, went very well. I think the worst part was getting the spinal anesthesia and the weird pressure feeling while they sewed the cervix and then tied the knot. I had minimal bleeding the day of and the day after. The doctor wrote a Rx for Tylenol with codeine but I thankfully did not have to use it. I had very minimal pain, and it was bearable and basically gone within a couple days. I stayed home from work and rested for six days. That really helped a lot. I was also given Metrogel vaginal cream to insert each evening. It's an antibiotic to help prevent infection. I still check my temperature when I start not feeling well. Thank goodness it's been OK.

I returned to work on Tuesday, 08.21.12. I felt really good. I must say, though, that toward the end of the day I realized I might have overdone it. I worked basically a full day and think that was too much for my first day back. I actually got really scared when I got home because my body just ached, and I was just praying the discomfort would go away soon. By Wed morning, I felt all better. So, I only worked five hours on Wed.

I went in this morning for my follow-up ultrasound. The tech was really nice and talked to me almost the entire time while doing the scan. My cervix was long (3.8cm) and closed. The babies are GREAT!!! Both have nasal bones, and the measurement of the folds behind the neck seemed to be fine, as well. These scans were done as part of the first trimester screening that is performed to give the parents the probability of the children having trisomy 13, 18, and 21.

While doing the scan, we were able to see the sex of one of the babies! Twin A is now known as baby boy! Baby B was harder to confirm. She even printed the scans and went to get the other tech to look at them and they both couldn't confirm. From one angle, it seemed like one sex, and from another angle it seemed like the other. So, we at least got the know one of the babies. We'll be able to confirm both at the 18-week anatomy scan in a few weeks☺. I forgot to mention that because my husband was not able to be there with me today (he got home at

4 a.m.), she didn't tell me the sex of the baby. The one she was able to confirm, she put in a sealed envelope and told me to open when I got home so I could share it with him. I thought that was really sweet of her. My husband liked that, too, as he woke up immediately when I got home (needed to stop by to change my bottoms) to find out how the appt went. So, needless to say, he was excited when we were able to find out the sex of at least one of the babies.

Since the scan to check the cervical measurement had to be done vaginally, I am experiencing a bit of discomfort down there. It seemed to have let up a bit since I used the restroom and emptied my bladder. I'm looking forward to going home in a couple hrs. so I can rest up a bit as it's been a long day for me already.

My husband and I are very thankful to the Lord our God for these miracles we've been blessed with. We're taking things one day at a time and as long as I do my part, the rest is up to God.

Monday, 09.03.2012 (15wk1d) — It's Labor Day. By the grace of God, we've made it to 15 weeks. There's only one more week until the next milestone, 16 weeks. I must say that I feel good. The only main ailment I can complain of is the pubic bone pain. It doesn't hurt from the outside. I get the pain on the inside of the pubic bone. So, I cannot even reach it if I wanted to in order to massage it or something. I have an OB appt on Friday so I will definitely bring it up to the doc then. In the meantime, I've been doing online research and there is actually a name for it. They say the cause is due to the ligaments stretching and the hormones causing softening of the bones/ligaments to make room for the growing uterus. When this happens, it causes the bone to be painful. I experience pain when trying to turn in bed, walking, getting in the car, etc. I was a bit relieved when I heard it was pretty normal. The downfall is that it's common in twins and really doesn't go away until after delivery of the babies. Besides that pain, I do not have any other real ailments. Since the cerclage, I do not feel pressure in the lower abdomen area like I felt in the last pregnancy. My back only aches once I've sat for too long, so I try to walk around for a few minutes as to not stay seated for long periods of time. I'm continuing to take things one day at a time until we deliver safe, healthy, and happy babies.

Wasn't Expecting This

As the pregnancy progressed, my work life did not let up. As per usual, things were busy, to say the least. It's now September and I have four cost reports due by October 31st. I am a planner, and hate to wait until the last minute to do anything. As such, I had everything under control with regards to the information needed from the various departments to file the reports. There were some final decisions that had to be made by management before submitting them officially.

As the time went on, we began discussing a baby shower. My husband was very adamant on me having one as I didn't get a chance to do so with the first pregnancy. I was reluctant to start planning because I felt I needed and wanted to wait until I was further along, just to be safe. On the flip side, waiting also ran the risk not being able to secure a venue location to have the shower because they need to be booked months in advance.

As my deadline got closer, I went in to work on a weekend to try and finish up the reports. I remember having to go in on Saturday, October 20th. As I prepared to leave the house, my mother-in-law said to me how beautiful I looked and how well I was carrying the babies. I was wearing blue jean shorts and flowy top. I smiled and thanked her. It was amazing because outside of normal pregnancy things, I was great.

My husband drove me to the office. As I was working, I started to not feel too well. I felt like there was pressure in my vaginal area. There was no pain but it felt like something heavy, lots of pressure. I then thought back to when I was in the shower and as I was washing my privates, I felt I touched something foreign. I didn't think much of it because I figured maybe my cervix was positioned lower and that was a stitch from the cerclage. As I began to feel bad, I thought of that and said, "I need not chance it."

I called my husband to pick me up. I didn't want to alarm him. While he was on his way, I called Dr. Yasin's office and weekend hotline. They advised me to come in to the hospital. Because I was already 20 weeks, they allowed me to go the pregnancy floor vs. the regular ER, thank God. When I arrived, after being checked in, the on-call doctor checked me. They explained that everything looked fine. The cervix was not open on physical exam and on ultrasound. Then Dr. Yasin called and spoke to me. He explained that, although everything looked OK, he was ordering for me to stay in the hospital for the weekend on bed rest where they could watch me actually be on bed rest vs. trusting me to do it at home. He said the pressure I was feeling was weird so it may be something starting that they just can't see yet.

I didn't freak out but thought it was a bummer. I immediately notified my manager that I was unable to finalize the reports because I am now in the hospital being watched but that I most likely would be discharged Monday, and we'd continue to from there. So, of course the worry and stress that comes with calling immediate family members and friends to tell them I'm in the hospital began to manifest. I was fine but having to tell them made me nervous because I knew it meant they'd now worry too. ☹

Let's Get Checked and Brace Yourself Again

Monday morning rolled around. Dr. Yasin came in very early to see me. I was happy to see him. He just gives off a sense of calm. Nonetheless, he had a student with him and asked my permission for him to be there. I was OK with that. So Dr. Yasin proceeded to check me and he was quiet. I immediately knew something was not right. He then called the student over and had him take a picture. Dr. Yasin then said, "Marline your cervix has opened up." I was shocked. I started crying immediately. How?

Why? I didn't do anything; I was here in bed all weekend. He explained that is exactly why he chose to have me stay because then they know they could try and pinpoint it without patient interference.

So, we asked what was next. I got back in to bed and they put me on the monitor again. Although I was not having contractions over the weekend, after being told my cervix was open, the contractions kept coming and wouldn't stop. Dr. Yasin explained that I had to remain calm because there is nothing he could do if I kept having contractions. He was tough when he needed to be. He said to me, "You were fine all weekend, and you get the news and now you're not, to the point that your body is reacting to these emotions. You must calm down, so the contractions can stop." I eventually did just that.

I became extra emotional because when all of this was happening was while I was 22 weeks along. This is the exact gestation point I was when I was losing our baby girl Angel. SO it REALLY HIT HARD.

It took a while for the contractions to calm down. Once they did, by later afternoon, it was too late to go for surgery. So, they gave me some meds, which I don't like because although they stop the contractions, they speed up my heart rate and affect my blood pressure — it's an awful feeling. Once I got that med and recouped from its side effects, I was good. Dr. Yasin came in and said, "Nothing to eat or drink after midnight because we're going in for an emergency cerclage in the morning." I was ready. I just knew it would fix the problem and I'd be on my way.

Tuesday morning, I get prepped and wheeled in to the operating room for surgery. My cervix had opened up 4cm. This is in spite of having a cerclage in place. That was just mind-boggling to me. Nonetheless, the surgery was a success. In the meantime, I was able to see the babies every day because they ordered ultrasounds to check on them before, during, and after the procedure. It was funny to see how Baby B (Kamden) was kicking his brother Baby A (Kason) even though they were in separate sacs. I thought the sacs would burst with all the activity and pressure I saw going on in there. Everyone assured me they'd be fine.

Now that the emergency cerclage was placed, I stayed in the hospital for observation. While at the hospital I had good and bad days emotionally. I had other friends who were also pregnant, so having them call to check in on me was great too. I also worked while in the hospital. Remember those reports that were days away from their deadline? Well, I had left them pretty much almost completed. There was simply one decision needed by management in order to finalize a particular cost center. I made notes and sent to my manager that covered where I left off, what was needed, etc. I felt bad because she had to cancel her Halloween trip with her daughter and granddaughter so she could finish these reports on time.

After about seven more days, I was cleared to go home on strict bedrest. Only one fast shower a day allowed and I could move from my bed to a recliner and back. Also, I could get up to go to the restroom and that was it. That is exactly what I did. One of my co-workers, Elizabeth, came to my house to get trained on a few things that she would handle while I was out.

One Step Forward and Two Steps Back

I then was scheduled to go for a follow-up appointment on Friday, 11.01, to see Dr. Y. At that appointment, he would check my cervix to ensure it was closed. Based on how that appointment went, we would determine if we'd book the venue for the baby shower.

While at the appointment, Dr. Yasin checked my cervix and again he was quiet. He kind of sighed and said, "OK guys." After only about two weeks since surgery, the cervix had opened again. I felt a wave of defeat come over me. My husband just looked at me. There were no words. He instructed us to go to the hospital across the street to be checked in. Now, we were going to stay there until the babies are born.

There was a lot of emotion going on. I remember all the departments coming in one after the other to talk to us about the options and the babies and me and this and that. Like ugh, please go away already. Dr. Yasin made sure I was given a great private room. The staff were a mess. Some of the nurses and PCAs were EXCELLENT. Others were just — no comment. Dr. Yasin was insistent on me making sure I spoke up when I needed something and not to be the "nice lady" because it can't be at the expense of saving my babies.

The Hospital is Now Home Again

Finally, after two more weeks in the hospital, numerous visits from family and friends, home-cooked meals being delivered, I was over it. I wanted to be home in my comfy bed but I knew this way was for the best. While there, I got an unexpected visitor, my dad. He came to visit with my mom. I was soooooo shocked, to say the least. We both began crying but before my dad could really show it, he just touched the end of my bed where I think he knew my feet to be and then stepped out of the room and stood right outside my door. It was very overwhelming but definitely a turning point in our relationship, at least for me and my outlook on where we stood.

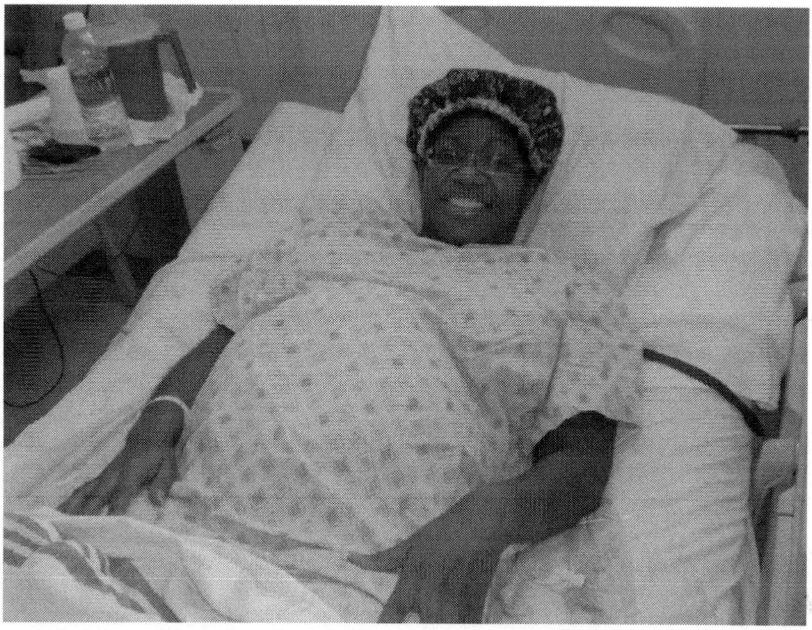

(Nov 2012 – Holtz Children's / Jackson Memorial Hospital, Miami, FL – 1 to 2 weeks prior to delivering the twins via emergency c-section. 26+1 weeks at delivery but belly measured 34 weeks)

It's important to support people when they're hospitalized because it's just a different kind of difficulty, almost, torturous experience for them while there, especially depending on why they're hospitalized. I have to say certain moments stood out to me while being in the hospital.

- My mom-in-law was sure to keep up with making my favorite foods and having my husband come and bring to me every day or every other day. She called every evening or morning to pray and reassure me everything would be OK. You could hear the worry and sometimes sadness in her voice but she tried her best to keep my spirits up.

- My sister, even though she worked a lot and had two jobs, made it her business to come visit whenever she was off. She would come by herself and on the weekends, she would bring my nieces and nephew. Seeing them always made my day and cheered me up. As my sister is a nurse, she had this calming directness about her in how she explained certain things to me that the medical staff would say. My hair was a mess because I couldn't get it done. She took out my extensions, sew-in for me, braided my real hair down and we put it in a bonnet for the remainder of the time I was in the hospital. That meant a lot because it reminded me of when she used to do my hair when I was a young girl. I loved how she braided my hair in cool styles back then because my mom only knew the regular styles with bows, ribbons and barrettes, no stylish braids. As a 4th and 5th grader, having her do my hair made me feel cool. So, her making sure my hair was at least presentable in the hospital meant everything to me!
- My friend Sonia had recently delivered my godson Kameron. So, she was not able to come and visit as she was on leave and had to care for her toddler daughter Kaelyn as well as a newborn. I can tell you our daily

phone dates kept me going. It was a breath of fresh air to look forward to our calls each day. If there was a time she didn't call me, I would call her to make sure she was OK as well. Although we never really talked about being in the hospital much, I knew she wanted to make sure I was OK and having our 'normal talk about everything talks' would help me feel better. It did. To give some history, Sonia and I would be on 2-3 hr long phone calls to catch up on things from the last time we spoke. If we actually saw each other, forget it, lol. Our husbands even knew to just kind of fall back when the two of us were on the phone 😊That was truly a great experience. I felt like we were in our own way helping each other get thru our new stages of life.

- My friend Maria was great. She didn't come often but we spoke all the time, very routinely. During one of our conversations I was telling her about my experience with the nursing staff and my care, and she felt horrible. She then reached out to her sister, Zsa, and they offered to come and help me where I lay in bed. I want to cry just thinking about it. I told them it was OK, but I truly appreciate them both extending help to me. One of the Sundays she visited with my godson Dorrien. I brought up needing a wax. I'm very hairy and also have what I call a 'female beard', lol. So what did she do? Yes, pulled out my tweezers — I had Kev bring them for me but didn't have the motivation or energy to do it myself — and she plucked out all of my beard hair. I was soooooo thankful and appreciative. It's something I will never forget. I get emotional whenever I think of it. Talk about a great friend and person. Forever grateful for her.

- My friend Julie and her mom visited on the Sunday right before I had the boys. I love to see Julie's mom. She is just so cute and caring. I don't mean to say cute in a bad way but rather the way she empathizes and takes on your feelings is amazing. Hearing her encouraging words that day even though I was feeling like crap was good for my mental health. It meant so much and helped a great deal.
- Jakisha, my friend Jakisha. She was my spiritual anchor during this time. We didn't see each other as often but my goodness did she keep the bible verses and prayers coming consistently. I am not sure what I would do without those faith-filled reminders. They mean more than she could ever imagine. There's nothing like a praying friend. All of our talks mainly focused on encouraging me and ensuring I stayed strong through this test because she knows I would pass it like I have all the others. ☺ That was our thing, taking tests, as she helped motivate me to get through my CPA testing, which was a bear. But she always reminds me

that with the Lord's grace, I did it! So she was steadfast in helping get thru again.

My cousins, friends, co-workers, work associates, family, EVERYBODY – too many to name, did their best to check in on me routinely while I was laid up in that hospital. Although on some days I did not feel like interacting, it is all the thoughts, texts, prayers, phone calls, visits that kept me going. I am FOREVER appreciative for them (Everyone and Everything)!

It's Go Time – The Babies Can't Wait

On Saturday, Nov 17th I started not to feel well in the evening. I just couldn't get comfortable. I felt like my bed all of a sudden was not comfortable; everything hurt. I told the nurse and spoke with the doctor and they gave me morphine. I was finally able to sleep around 2 a.m. that night. Sunday, Nov 18th the next day rolled around and after church more people came to visit. Both my mom-in-laws, brother-in-law, friend Julie and her mom, and more were like, "You don't look too good, so ask for some Tylenol." I finally did that, and it took the edge off but I was still uncomfortable.

The nurses put me on the monitor to see if I was having contractions since I was so uncomfy. They picked up nothing on the monitor. After everyone left, the nurse came in to check me and found I was having contractions after the monitor moved and shifted position. They immediately checked me and found I was dilated 4, almost 5cm.

They immediately called the doctor and he had them prep the operating room for an emergency C-section. Dr. Yasin must've flown there. He got there in no time. By the time he came and they had raced me to the operating room, I was already 6cm dilated. I remember them telling me not to push. I did not have the urge to push, thank God. All of the pain was in my back. It was horrific. The back pain was unbearable. It was as though someone was taking a crowbar and prying both sides open and apart. My God.

Before you know it, the babies were delivered. They were born at 12:58 a.m. and 12:59 a.m. on Monday, Nov 19th 2012! I remember he asked if I had specific names for the babies based on A or B. I said yes so he told the team to label them correctly, LOL. Kason, Baby A, came out first. After a few seconds, he started crying. It was the most beautiful, faint yet strong cry I heard. Then Baby B, Kamden, was delivered. I did not remember hearing his cry until after they took him over to the side and I guess were working on him, and then I heard the slight whimper. It was music to my ears.

Too Afraid to be Happy

I was then taken to recovery. I remember being itchy. The nurse must've given me too many meds to combat that because I had a difficult time waking up in recovery. Dr. Yasin wanted me up and alert before I could be taken to my actual room. I remember my first set of visitors were my mom, sister, and brother-in-law, Choubert T.

My phone did not stop ringing. The texts were coming and coming. They were from family and friends sending congratulations about the birth of the twins. I was confused. I did not feel happy. Why was everyone else happy? How do I even know these babies were going to survive? I can't celebrate yet. They were born at 26 weeks and 1 day. That's just too early. I had all of these thoughts going through my head.

My mom and sister got to go to the NICU to see the babies. They were able to see Kason but Kamden was having a procedure done so they couldn't see him clearly. It was tough. The next day my baby brother Berny and Jasmine, big and pregnant as she was due in less than 2 months, came by to visit as well. It was great because while they were there, the nurses wanted me to get up and walk and go to the bathroom for the first time. OMG, I thought I was going to die. It was brutal. Thank goodness they were there because both Berny and Jasmine literally and physically helped me out of bed and get to the bathroom as well. That was the day I also got to see the boys for the first time. Kev was working, so Berny was there to wheel me to the NICU. The nurse had a bit of a time pronouncing the last name. I then told her to think of Duracell battery and she'd get it — Duroseau. She loved that idea and everyone that came by she told them how to pronounce the boys' names. She even said, they're strong and just like the battery they'll keep going and charging through 😊.

Finally, the day came, two days later, Wednesday, and I had begged Dr. Yasin to go home. I didn't want to spend Thanksgiving in the hospital. So we planned that if I used the restroom (had a bowel movement) and got up to walk by Wednesday, he would agree to discharge me because I had been here for so long already.

I was happy to be home for Thanksgiving. I felt guilty leaving the twins there ☹. However, after that day, the new life and routine began for our family.

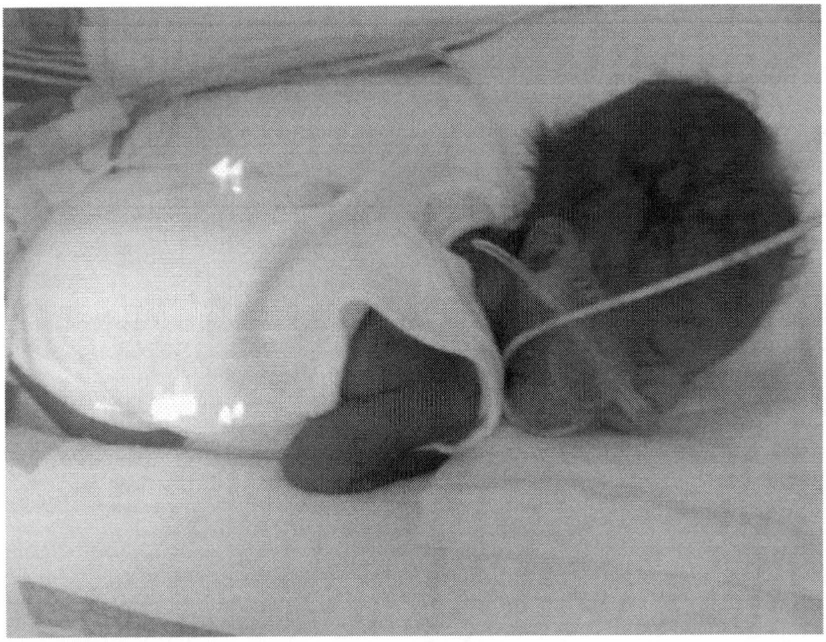

(Holtz Children's NICU @ Jackson Memorial Hospital, Miami, FL - Baby A – Kason – Born 2lbs – on cannula oxygen, tube for feeding)

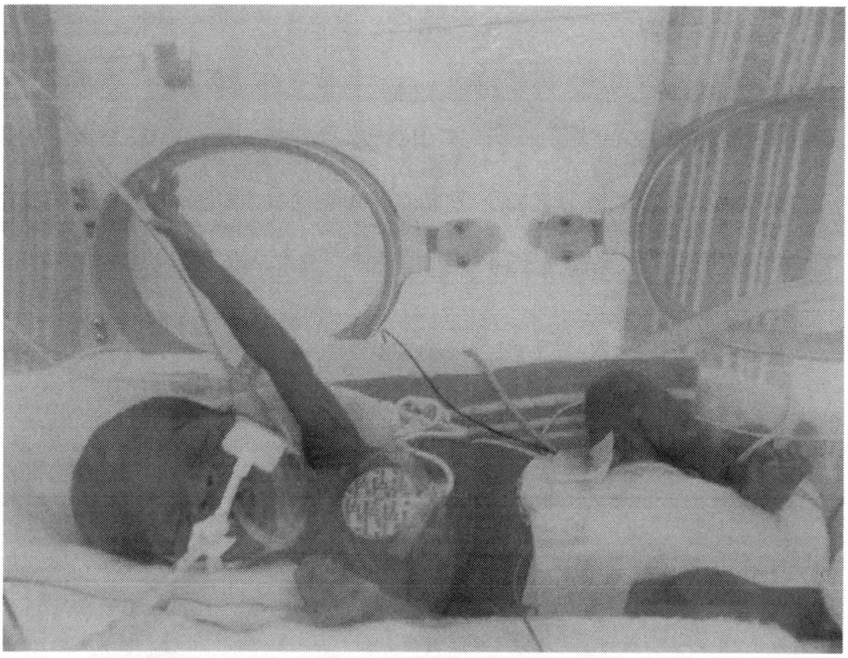

(Holtz Children's NICU @ Jackson Memorial Hospital, Miami, FL - Baby B – Kamden – Born 1lb 12ozs – on central line intubation for oxygen; tube feeding. Our little fighter raising his hand in power!)

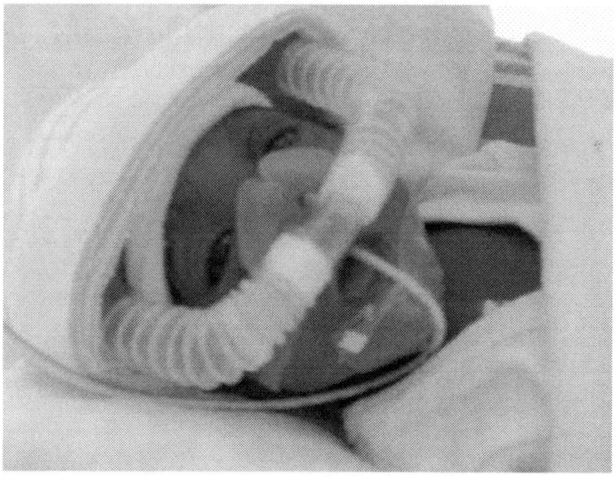

(Holtz Children's NICU Miami, FL - Baby A – Kason – c-pap for oxygen; tube feeding.)

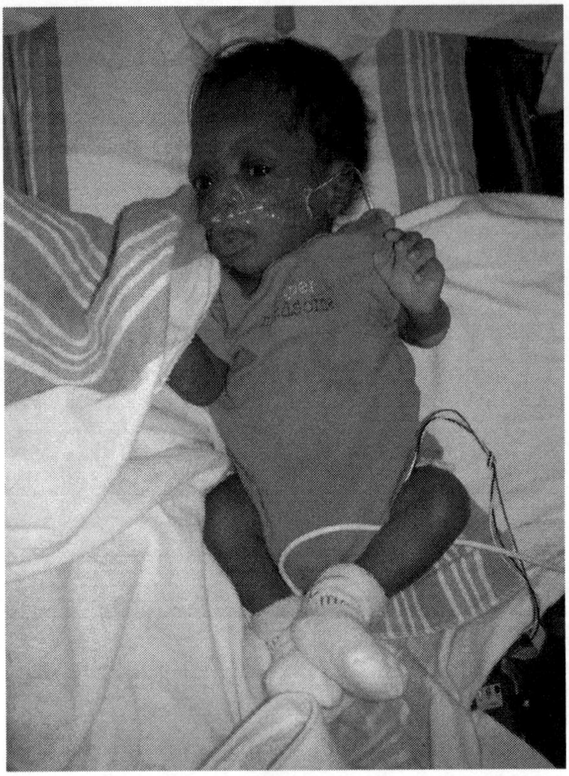

(Holtz Children's NICU Miami, FL - Baby B – Kamden – cannula for oxygen; preemie outfit and socks)

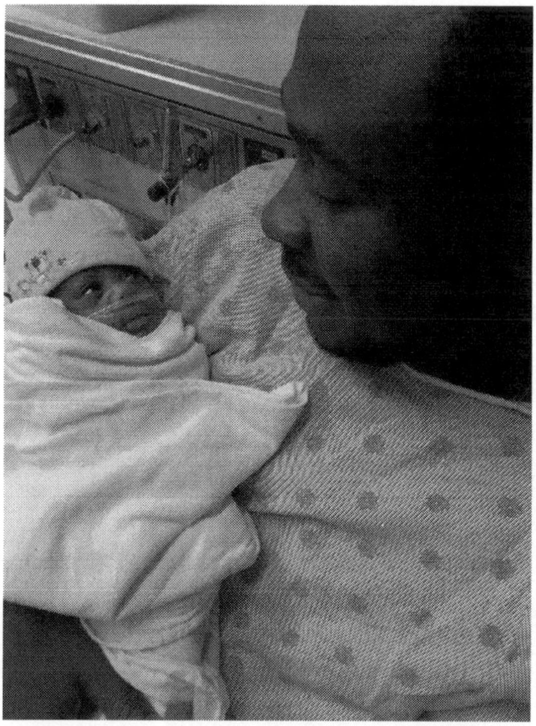

(Holtz Children's NICU Miami, FL - Baby A – Kason – bonding w/daddy)

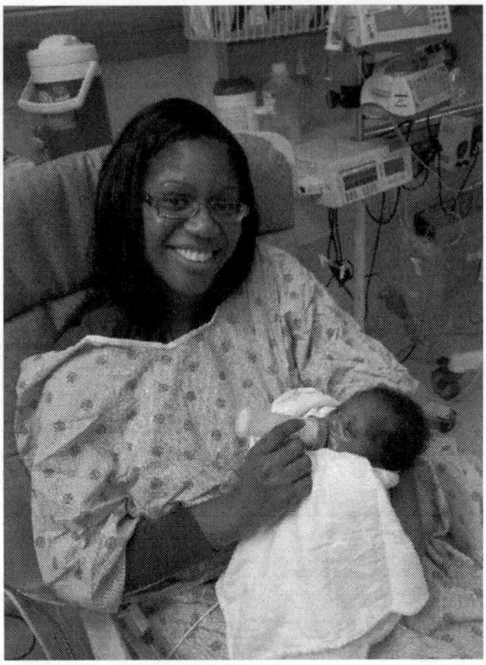

(Holtz Children's NICU Miami, FL - Baby B – Kamden – breastmilk bottle feeding w/mommy)

Answered Prayer

We asked, prayed, prepped, and waited for a blessing. This cycle had repeated itself year after year. When finally, our prayers and requests were answered, there ensued a quiet stage, a wondering stage, a confused stage, "What do we do now? Are we actually able to even handle these double blessings, this new situation we were just gifted? Everything will be OK though, right?"

I have to tell you, things were very hectic, to say the least, after welcoming these babies into the world. I never thought that after fighting so hard, we'd have to continue to fight. The battle wasn't over simply because we won.

Needless to say, life completely changed. In a way, I guess I expected it to change but it didn't happen in the manner in which I thought it would. I was still a career professional and had to juggle work. I was still a wife and had to ensure my husband was OK and the household responsibilities didn't fall to the wayside. I was still Marline and had to find a way to not totally lose myself. Yet, I also thought, how do I make room to do all of these things and take care of two helpless, fragile little people who were totally dependent on me?

After being born via emergency C-section, the babies spent (only days shy of) four months in the NICU. It was rough! There's something very emotionally devastating about giving birth and not leaving the hospital with your child(ren). Having to go home without the twins immediately resulted in me reliving my experience almost a year earlier with Angel. It's just awful. So many thoughts ran through my head — will my babies make it? Are they in pain? Why is this happening? I won't be able to survive this if anything happens to them. Please let them be OK. These thoughts circled in my mind like a merry go round; over and over again.

Now We're Living the NICU Life

While in the NICU, I was able to establish a daily routine that helped me get my head on track as it related to my thoughts. I wasn't physically able to go to my therapy sessions but all of my team of docs checked in on me periodically. This included my reproductive endocrinologist (Dr. Hoffman), my acupuncturist (Dr. Duro), and my therapist (Dr. Cheryl Gotthelf). That helped a lot.

On a given day, I would wake and then pray. Next up, shower and have a hearty breakfast, which my mom-in-law made. After eating, I'd sit in the family room or the guest bedroom and pump. Once done, I'd switch out the pump parts for cleaned sterilized ones. I'd prep the bag containing the breast pump, pump parts, milk bags, change of clothes for the kids — we'd bring in preemie clothes for them to wear — pack a lunch and then head off to work.

Two weeks after giving birth, I went back to work. It was more to ease my mind to avoid idle thoughts that ran wild. Also, there is always work to do. I was heavily involved in a project that we needed to try and finalize by a certain date. Plus, why not go back to work while the babies were in the NICU and I could take time off once they're released to actually be home with them on maternity leave?

So once I packed everything up after pumping, I headed to my office. I'd work from about 10:30 a.m. until 3 p.m. While still at work, I would pump, bag, and store the milk. If time permitted, I would quickly eat the lunch I brought. Around 3:00/4:00 p.m., depending on how the day went, I would leave the office and head to the NICU.

Once at the NICU, I would sit with both babies. Oftentimes, they progressed together to where they'd be side by side or in close proximity of each other in the NICU. There were lots of ups and downs and emergency procedures, blood transfusions, spinal taps, etc., during their stay there. So on some visits, for days or weeks at a time, I'd have to split my time between the boys because they weren't in the same area. That was tough because I wanted to be there for both of them equally.

One plus that came out of going to the NICU daily is the friendships and bonds that form between the moms, dads, and extended families as everyone is in the same boat as it relates to hoping and praying our kids make it through. I must also tell you there is something very humbling about witnessing some parents lose their precious babies while in NICU. This just reminded me of how lucky and blessed we were and to not take each day for granted.

I usually left the NICU around 11:30 p.m. to 1:00 a.m. because by then I needed to pump. Usually I also waited for shift change and bath time, when they got older, to allow for smooth transitions between staff and the babies' care.

After two months in the NICU, we felt comfortable enough to take the advice of family and friends to actually reschedule and have the twins' baby shower. It was awesome and truly a blessing. They even looked good enough two days before the shower to take nice pictures of them. We created a collage and displayed these pics at the shower. I had never been to a shower for a non-pregnant person so I was reluctant to do it. Thank goodness we did because it made everyone very happy.

Throughout all of this, my husband still worked the night shift. Well, he started work at 5:00 p.m. and usually didn't leave until 3:30 a.m. That is on a good and normal day. During busy season, he'd leave work well into the next morning. So, he was only able to see the babies on the weekends for the most part.

They're Finally Coming Home

The day came when the boys got to come home. Kamden came home on Friday, 03.08.13, evening. Kason came home the following Monday, 03.11.13, three days later. They had been scheduled to come home together. However, Kason was scheduled for an inguinal hernia surgery for Tuesday, 03.05.13, but his surgeon became sick so his procedure was cancelled and rescheduled for Friday, 03.08.13. Because he needed to be watched for three days post op, he was not able to come home the same day of surgery. There was no longer any medical reason to hold Kamden. Thus, he was discharged on the same evening Kason had surgery. It was almost as though they knew they were leaving each other. That was an emotional three days apart but, yes, Kason did great post-op and was reunited with his brother three days later.

Now the fun began. One benefit of having only one baby home was we were able to kind of establish a little bit of a routine with Kamden. When Kason came a few days later, we just added one more to the mix. 😊

Things got very tricky once life with the twins became our new normal. In order to maintain a sense of sanity, I had to turn off the chip in my head that called for perfection in everything. That just couldn't happen. I had to learn to do the best I could with what I had. In hindsight I can write about that now, but that was not my reality at the time. I was very frustrated and upset that things were not unraveling as I had thought.

My husband still worked overnight. So there was not much assistance from him when it came to caring for the boys during those early years. During the day, he slept. Of course it's normal, but I just couldn't help but feel resentment toward him because it was not fair he got to get uninterrupted sleep and I didn't. I have to also say I had lots of help with the twins. My mother-in-law still lived with us. My stepmom-in-law came over every other evening after work and on the weekends. My mom would come over weekly. They each handled and were responsible for something as it related to helping take care of the house, the babies, me, and my recovery, running errands etc. I was supposed to use that time to rest and sleep, but of course, I did not. All of that just catches up to you at some point.

My Brother and Cousins were My Keepers

My 32nd birthday was fast-approaching when the boys were released from the NICU. It was about 2 weeks away I think. Of course there was no celebrating a birthday for me. I was engrained in all things baby. Two nights before my birthday my cousin Laurie J had worked it all out to be with me to help since the boys were now home. She was excited about coming over to help. Needless to say, my dearest cousin Laurie got a run for her money, LOL. She stayed over 3 days and 3 nights. Poor thing, she got no sleep with those twins. I felt safe and comfortable having her there to watch the kids and I actually got about 5 hours of sleep on the nights she was there. She was terrific but it was a lot. I am so grateful for her doing that because at that time, Laurie's children were babies too. Three of them. It was selfless of her to leave Joshua, Jeremiah and Julia just to come and help me. I will never ever forget that.

On the actual day of my birthday, the boys had their 1st apt at the pulmonologist. They also had a pediatrician apt because their reflux was starting up. There was also another apt, which I cannot remember but we had like 3 appts on that day. Laurie was a trooper in that she helped get the kids ready, helped pack their bags, bottles, etc and we were out. We spent the entire day on the road with the boys going from doctor to doctor as scheduled that day. Because it was my birthday, she insisted on stopping by a popular Haitian Restaurant we both liked and she purchased dinner for me. It was such a thoughtful gesture. Once we got home, she helped me get the kids in and settled and helped grandma wash and fold their clothes. I remember that day like it was yesterday. I have to tell you I remember when her husband came to pick her up, she looked exhausted. I know he was probably wondering what I did to his wife, smh. I am forever grateful for my cousin (more like sister) Laurie 😊.

Another memory I still hold dear during this time after having the boys is me trying to regain some sense of normalcy as it relates to just feeling like myself and doing things I used to do. My friend Maria and sisters-in-law Anne and Jasmine set up a birthday outing for me a few weeks after the boys came home. I was not really up for it, but they insisted we celebrate. Ugh, everyone knows I am a birthday junkie. We dined at Brio Italian restaurant. It was nice to be out and enjoy the company of other women, my friends. However, the entire time I was thinking about the boys at home. The highlight of that outing for me was when the ladies presented me with a gift during our lunch. I immediately got emotional because I don't like to receive gifts; I prefer to give. I opened the envelope and it was a significant donation to the March of Dimes on behalf of Kason and Kamden and their time in the NICU. They were right, they knew I'd cry and I did. It was one of the most thoughtful gifts I had received. The

March of Dimes supports premature babies and helps the NICU's care for them. It was simply beautiful.

There was no way I could have gotten through those first few months of having the boys home without my brother Berny as well. Remember, Jasmine was pregnant too and my niece Bailey was both in January, 2 months after the twins. Berny worked 2nd shift at his company. Thus, he usually got off of work around 11:30pm/midnight. I have to tell you, without me asking, just because I didn't really think to anyway as to not bother or impose, he came over every night after leaving work. (I'm tearing up as I remember this). He did not come over on Fridays because at the time my husband was off on Fridays. Berny was there from about 11:45pm/12:15am until about 3:30am, sometimes past 4am when my husband came home from work to basically relieve him. At this time, he too had a little baby at home too. I was taken aback and just overwhelmed with gratitude. He said he wanted to help because he knew I wasn't really sleeping and with him there, I could at least sleep and he would watch and take over the 2am feeding for the boys. I didn't wake my mom-in-law during the night as she was up all day with the kids. Berny knew I worked during the day and was up with the kids at night as my husband had to work. It was just the most thoughtful act ever. Jasmine and Anne even came over on the weekends with their babies to help keep me company. My siblings and I had babies in 2012, it was crazy (Narvens, Sydney, Kason, Kamden, Bailey - 5 cousins within weeks of each other). Berny was a life saver during this time for me and I will never forget it. I appreciate Jasmine for understanding and being supportive of this well. As luck would have it though, just a years later, they would have their own set of twins (Brent and Bryson) 😊

Some people that were close to me really stepped in to help me throughout the various stages of this journey. There is just not enough time or space to express all the gratitude I have for every single person that, in one way or another, who helped us. I am forever grateful to everyone 😊.

My cousin Charlene and I pretty much grew up together. I remember my aunt and uncle stopping by our house on their way home from the hospital after she was born. I was excited to run downstairs to see the new baby. She has just always been special to me. As we grew up we saw each other all time, almost every weekend. When our two families got together, she and I were the only girls so naturally we were together. When together, we talked about life, played with our hair (but was sure to put it back how it was because our moms were not with the idea of messing up our hair, lol), listened to and danced to music.

Our close relationship continued as we grew up through the years. When going through my struggle, she was there. She was not aware of the behind the scene details but she was there. I remember her visits to the hospital when I was pregnant with Angel and after I lost her. She kept me and all the visitors entertained. I remember her hitting it off with my sister-in-law

Nadia. They were cutting up in the hospital room. They may not have known it, but it was exactly what I needed. [Charlene kept the laughs coming and Nadia made sure I ate. Now that I think of it, Nadia always made it her business to make sure I eat when she attended any event I was having, lol. She reminded me I could not keep running around and not eat. She even does this 'til today! I love Nadia dearly!]

Even though I was sad after losing Angel, Charlene kept our standing Friday night date night. She was just there. I then became pregnant with the twins and even though I didn't tell her right away, she was there to support me. As I got further along in the twin pregnancy, she was on top of the 'checklists.' She planned our shopping trips that consisted of picking up last minute items for the boys. She helped me plan out and arrange the nursery. I remember she even helped pick out the boys nursery rug on our trip to Target one Saturday afternoon. She was just there.

After having the boys, needless to say I was having a hard time just even existing and adjusting to everything. Charlene still came over on Friday nights to help me with them and to just be there for me. I enjoyed giving her love, friendship and life advice during our talks. Kev traveled out of town a few times after I had the twins. Charlene is the one who went with me on Saturday pediatrician visits with the twins. Remember, I went nowhere alone with the kids. Because she was there, she helped me get them in an out of the car, up and down elevators, she pushed the boys' limo aka the double stroller. She was just there.

Jumping ahead a bit, when pregnant with our KB, Charlene was there. She and my niece Beatrice spear-headed the preparations for him. They came over on a Saturday afternoon and cleaned my entire room, cleared out the nursery by organizing gifts, etc. and rearranged my custom closet to ensure everything was in order and ready for the baby. That same Saturday morning we went shopping and she had her 'checklist' to make sure I also got the items I needed for myself – pajamas, robes, etc. for after the baby arrived. Charlene was and is just always there.

I look forward to the day when she has her 'it happened' moments. I cannot wait to just be there for her as we continue our cousin/sistership. I'm not sure what I would have done without her help, love and support – no questions, no explanations – she was just always there! 😊

I could write a whole book on married life, mom life, and woman's life after babies. As a matter of fact, stay tuned for that. That is just too much to unpack right now in this purpose.

Thank goodness for my company. They supported me on this journey from the beginning. When planning to have a baby and it doesn't happen the natural way, it takes lots of time, money, and flexibility as it relates to your schedule. Because I had been with my company about 10 years at this time, they were very understanding, helpful, and accommodating during this whole ordeal. Now that doesn't make it easy, but knowing I had the opportunity and flexibility to come and go, change my schedule, rearrange deadlines, and still meet my job requirements helped me through this extremely! In my position, not doing my job effectively or timely meant significant financial consequences to the organization. So, again I say, it wasn't easy because not being able to dedicate a full typical structured 40+ hours to my work brought on additional stress and worry in addition to juggling this new life and responsibilities.

From 2013, when the boys came home from NICU, until about 2016, it was non-stop appointments and doctor visits. They had weekly physical therapy appointments; monthly, then eventually quarterly cardiologist appointments; and ophthalmologist appointments to make sure their eyes were developing as they should. During flu season, the boys had monthly pulmonology appointments to receive a SYNAGIS injection so they did not develop respiratory syncytial virus (RSV), which could result in their death as micro preemies. That was a scary thought as many preemies have long-lasting effects from under-developed lungs. The pediatrician also wanted to see them monthly to ensure they were growing well and to help manage and treat their acid reflux.

The twins dealt with acid reflux horribly for a full year after coming home. So on top of all of that, it was hard to feed them because they didn't seem to be able to keep anything down. The boys had day-long evaluation appointments to ensure they were meeting milestones and not be developmentally delayed. Those appointments were grueling in the sense that they lasted almost the entire day and the kids became cranky. I am sure I am leaving some out but these appointments stand out the most.

I was never alone with the kids. Although they were mine and I knew how to deal with kids, these weren't normal kids, at least to me. I was afraid. So I was lucky to always have someone with me to go to these appointments and be at home.

I Think I Got It – New Normal

I can tell you that once the kids turned three, in late 2015, things sort of changed a lot. I became more sure of myself as a mom. The boys had met and surpassed their milestones. They were doing well in day care and were then placed in actual elementary school in the PK–3 program for further communication developmental delay assistance.

Once I gained some of my confidence back, I was able to have serious conversations with my husband about my feelings and everything that had transpired over the past three years. During this time, I had returned to therapy and Dr. Gotthelf helped me to find my foundation and center again. This enabled me to step right back in to all of my self-inflicted perfection roles while adding on the responsibilities the boys now brought.

Life with the boys became cooler and easier. My husband and I were back in a more normal space with our relationship, friendship, and marriage. That meant a lot to me. It also helped in my getting back to normal. As the boys got older, it was easier for my husband and me to travel with them, take them out to restaurants, just live life. I was able to start exercising, which I enjoyed, with my co-worker friends as accountability partners. I lost all the weight from the twins and was in great shape. I was content with how life was going.

I am not sure how I/we made it through those complicated times. It is only by the grace of God things got better. We just have to be ready for what we ask for. This goes for every aspect of asking for blessings. Whether it be educational, career, personal, family, etc., when you are granted your wish — think about if you can actually handle it. Do you really know what you're asking for? As a faith-filled person, I quickly began to live and experience what people say — sometimes you have to wait for your blessing because you have to be ready. You're being prepped and primed for what's to come. Once it does come, you'll be strong enough to go through it and have your testimony or happy ending when it's all said and done.

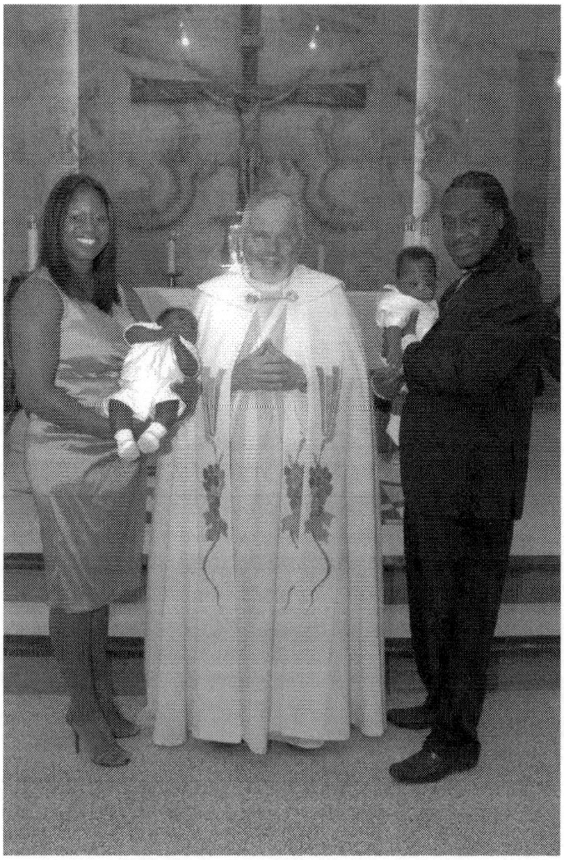

(May 2013 - Church of the Visitation of the Blessed Virgin Mary, Miami, FL – Fr. Curtis Kiddy at Kason and Kamden's baptism)

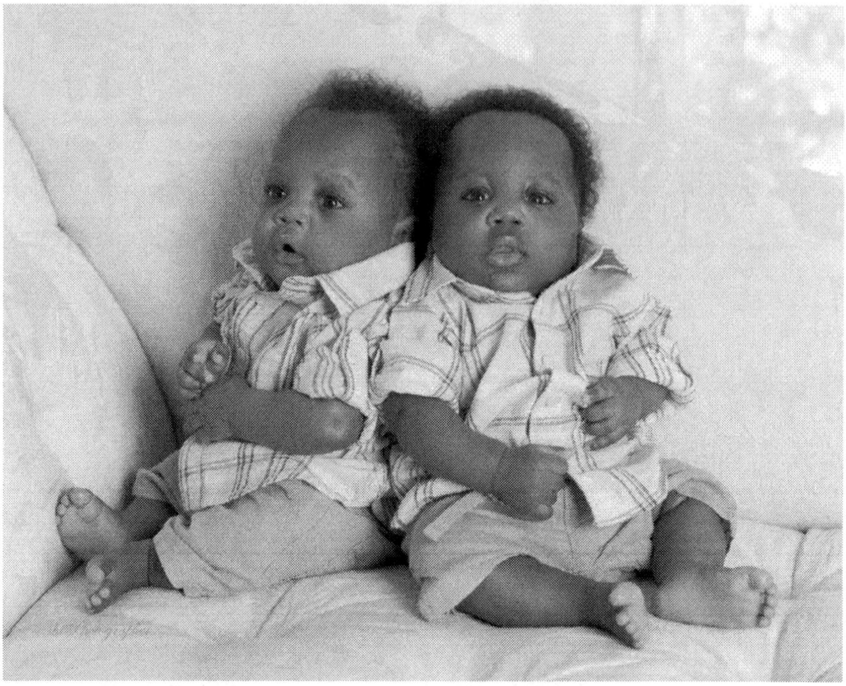

(June 2013 – DD Photographer, Ft Lauderdale, FL – Photo Shoot for Kason and Kamden since I missed out on my scheduled maternity shoot.)

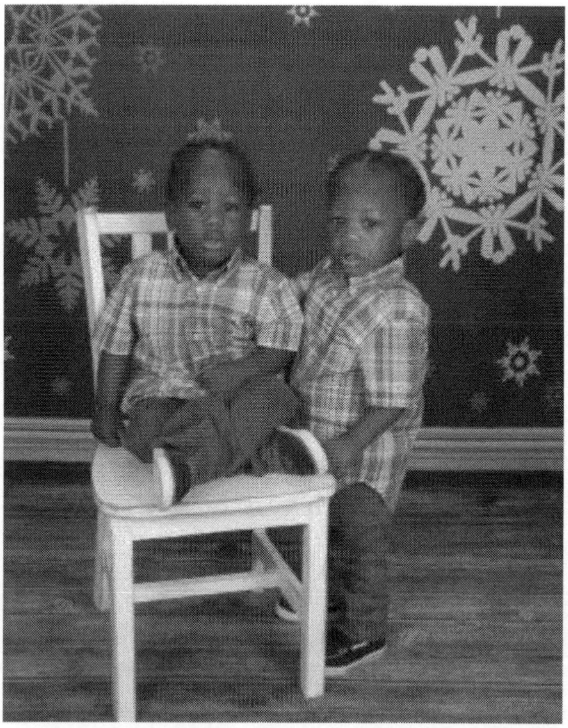

(Oct 2015 Wee Ones Day Care, Hollywood, FL – Kason and Kamden at school picture day.)

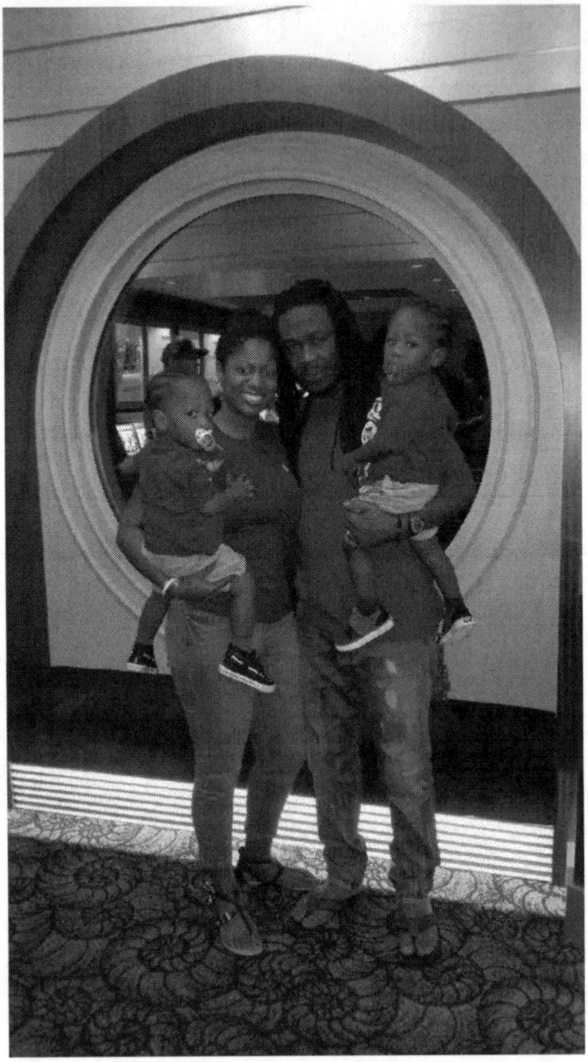

(Nov 2014 Disney Cruise – 1st time traveling with the twins. They loved the pacifiers!)

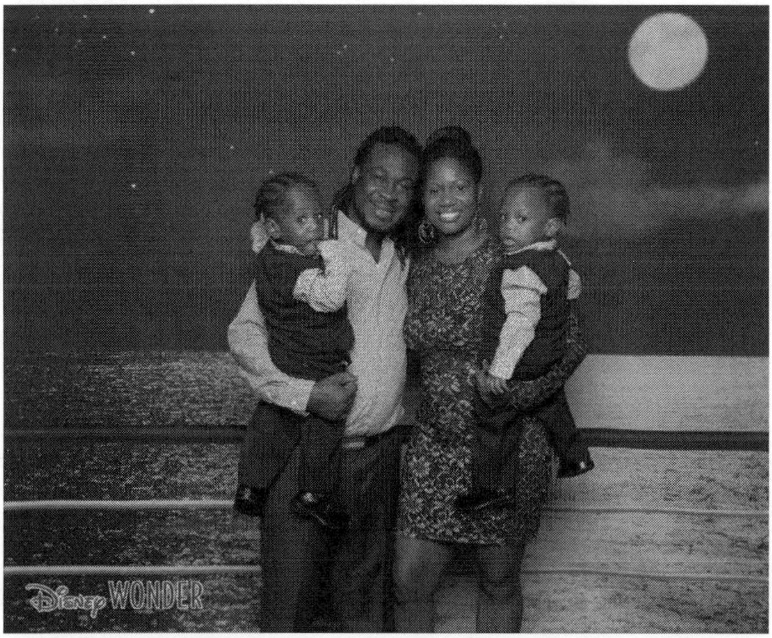

(Nov 2014 – Disney Cruise Pictures on Formal Night. We looked good but I remember so much worry and anxiety behind my smile)

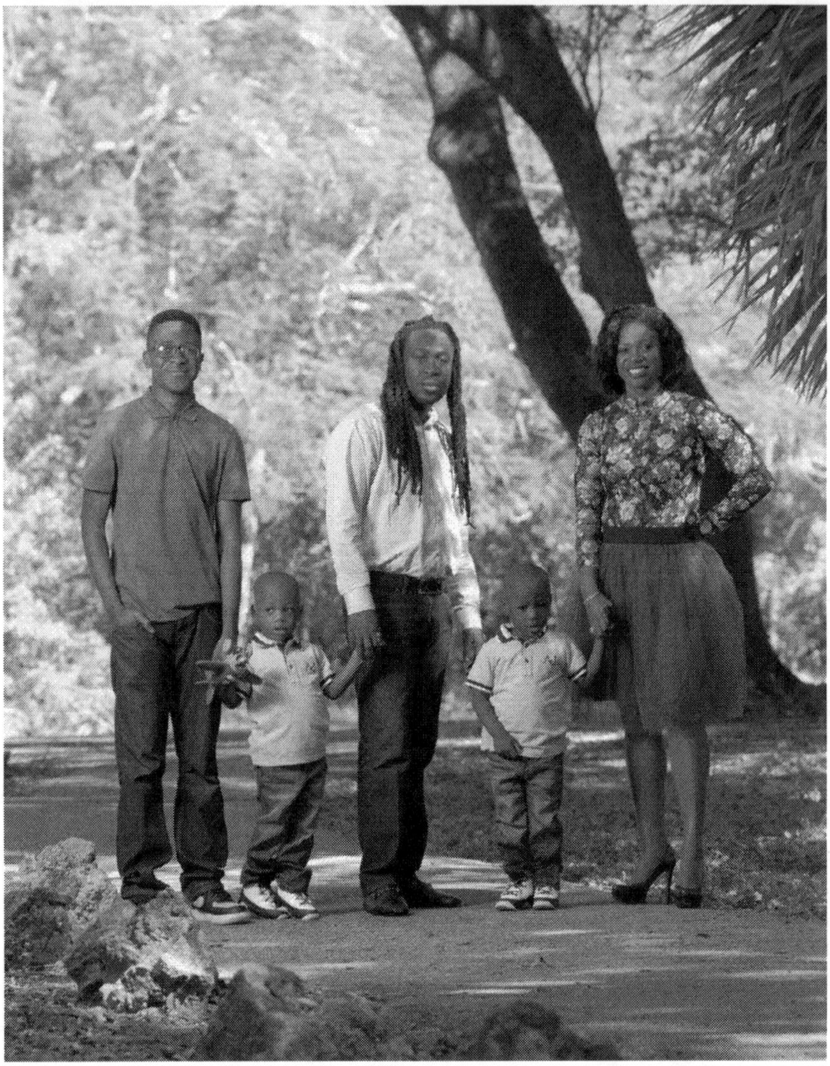

(Jan 2017 – Treetops Park, Davie, FL - Birthday Photoshoot for Richard, turned 21, and the twins, turned 4. Confidence was alive behind my smile now!)

New Normal

What About Doing It Again?

Almost immediately after giving birth, I wanted to have another "normal" baby right away. I felt like this until the boys were about two. I was not happy about the physical aspect of doing it again but these were the emotional thoughts I was dealing with. I had lots of guilt as I thought it was my fault them being born early. I do not think I actually wanted more kids at the time; I was trying to fill an emotional void.

Slowly but surely we gave more and more thought to possibly expanding the family. In order to do so, we gave considerable thought to the possibility of losing another pregnancy or even having a baby go through the NICU again due to my weakened cervix. As a way to avoid potentially losing another baby, I had to get my cervix 'fixed' if I even wanted to entertain this idea of expanding the family. We looked into the Transabdominal Cerclage (TAC) options again, after originally doing so and researching in 2014.

I wanted to have the TAC surgery after I had already gotten pregnant. I felt the only reason I was doing it was for a baby. So, if I didn't get pregnant then I wouldn't need to get it. After having three consultations with the doctors, we decided to do it before trying again. Dr. Haney was one of the pioneer doctors based out of Chicago. Dr. Leroy Charles was one of the laparoscopic method pioneer doctors in West Palm Beach. Finally,

Dr. Ricardo Estape was the leading DaVinci Robot doctors in Miami. All of them were specialists for the TAC. They felt although I needed to do IVF to get pregnant each time, when I did it, it worked. So, they pushed me to have the TAC before because, like my husband, they felt if IVF worked before, it would work again. So there was no need to add extra risk to having surgery while pregnant. I ultimately decided to go with Dr. Ricardo Estape for the TAC. After also consulting with Dr. Hoffman, I was then ready to start again.

All TAC'd Up – Let's Get Back to It

Journey to Frozen Embryo Transfer (FET)

Friday — September 9, 2016

I decided a couple of days ago to pick back up with my writing and journaling. Things are extremely busy for me now. Between work, the boys, family, trying to have a personal life — I'm swamped.

I just had a bout of nausea — ugh — never want to feel like that again if I can help it, LOL!

Friday — February 10, 2017

After healing from the TAC surgery, I wanted to start journaling again. The plan was start at the beginning of the FET cycle in Sep 2016 but I ultimately stopped just as soon as I started. There was just too much going on.

I can explain that the FET cycle is much less intrusive than going through IVF with a fresh cycle. With the FET cycle, there are no stimulation medications and no egg retrieval. Instead, there are some meds in the beginning of the cycle, including those to suppress ovulation and then an embryo transfer.

The cycle was actually a smooth one — again, much easier process than the fresh cycle. I had the TAC placed back on July 27, 2016. As mentioned previously, it was done by Dr. Estape via DaVinci Robot. The procedure went extremely well too, thank God. So I feel "fixed."

Not sure if I wanted to go at IVF again but being that I now have this permanent cerclage I feel it's only right and a sign that I try again. My husband agreed, mainly because he spear-headed campaign new baby Duroseau, so here we are.

Back to the FET. I wrote down all of my symptoms post transfer so I'll try and insert them in here when I have a chance. <>. When it was time to go in for the transfer, I was able to get my acupuncture session in early that morning. The clinic was gracious enough to rearrange the schedule so I could be later in line. When Crystal came in with the picture of our one embryo, I was overwhelmed with emotion. I dreaded that whole morning the possibility of receiving a phone call saying the embryo did not thaw well or arrested after thaw or something morbid along those lines. However, the little guy made it so we were thankful.

She did say, though, that the quality/grade was not that great. I was taken aback by that since I know that only strong embryos make it to the freezing stage. I had faith nonetheless that all would work out.

Now you no longer have to wait in the bed for 30 minutes post transfer before getting up to use the restroom and insert the progesterone. That was definitely something new. The Valium hit me almost immediately. I forgot to ask Dr. Barrionuevo what my lining was prior to the transfer. I was thinking it but couldn't mouth the words to ask. Five days before the transfer, my lining came back at like 6. So Nurse Nadia called in a script for Estrace tablets that I was to insert vaginally for five days to get the lining thicker. That kind of bummed me out a bit but when she looked back at my two prior cycles, my lining wasn't much better at this stage, so they felt that it was OK to add the Estrace and go from there.

I mentioned Dr. Barrioneuvo again. Of course we all felt great that it was he who did both successful transfers so that was a wonderful thing!

Everything went well post transfer. I was waiting for certain signs to compare to previous cycles. I think I'm a special case though because both prior cycles were so different. It was difficult to try and compare to this one. I did have some tell-tale symptoms like elevated heart beat or shortness of breath. I was very hungry a few days before test day. We were at work on hurricane watch and scarfed down lunch earlier than usual and had a big breakfast. A little while later I was hungry again. I also had episodes of heightened smell — both times I'd randomly get hit with the smell of like raw metal/blood. It was very weird and strong. The Monday and Wednesday before the test day (Sat) I just knew my cycle was coming. I felt very wet down there like I had just started my period. This happened very early in the morning while still in bed. I ran to the restroom both times and nothing. Ugh, it was an awful feeling.

I also got a few long naps in. One week before test day (Sat), I felt extremely tired and sleepy. I went to acupuncture in the morning, but I was unable to do anything else. I slept for hours and didn't think I'd feel well enough or rested enough to get up. I normally fight my sleep by watching TV, but no, I was out for the count. Kev took the boys for haircuts so they were out of the house for a few hours. He then took them to Chuck E. Cheese and then his dad's house. I went down maybe around 2 and didn't get back up again until almost 8 p.m. Then I jumped up feeling great and wanted IHOP pancakes, LOL. It was delicious.

I had that same urge to nap two days before test day. We got off of work early due to the hurricane and I went home and was knocked out. I didn't have any implantation bleeding this time, although maybe three days or so post transfer I had a light pink stain when I went to the restroom. It definitely wasn't there in the morning, rather a later afternoon pee session.

When It Rains It Pours

The worst part was the waiting. Original test day was Friday, 10.07.16, but due to the hurricane, it was changed to Saturday, 10.08.16. In the midst of all of this, Kason was sick and had to have surgery. ☹ He was having some pain in his leg one morning. After giving him some Tylenol he felt better so he went to school. The next day he woke up crying due to the pain in his leg. Kev and I took him to the ER. We found out he had some weird puss-filled cyst like thing in his lower hip area. At one point, they thought it was rheumatoid arthritis but thank goodness, it wasn't. After an x-ray and ultrasound, the ER Doctor used a huge syringe to obtain a sample of the fluid. As a mom, it was hard to watch that procedure. Although he was given a sedative, you can tell he was in pain. After giving him another dose of meds, they were able to obtain their sample. The testing and culture revealed It was highly infected and needed to be removed from that hip/leg joint immediately. So, Kason had the surgery that same day and was admitted to the hospital.

Kason was discharged on the following Monday. The embryo transfer was scheduled for the next day, Tuesday. It had been 6 days since he was in the hospital. During those 6 days, I had to give myself the necessary injections and insert my suppositories daily, as instructed by Dr. Hoffman. It was a very hectic time to say the least. After the transfer and during the two week wait, I had to run around with Kason to post-op appointments, etc.

Needless to say, it was not a successful cycle. I received notice that I was pregnant. I was pregnant again. My HcG Beta was a bit low so doctors said, "we're cautiously optimistic." Unfortunately, we suffered an early miscarriage. It was extremely devastating. I took it very hard. I cried the entire rest of the weekend. Still, I tried to keep faith alive that somehow the numbers would start rising, maybe it was a late implantation. But no, definitely not the case. I had to do a repeat hCG and it confirmed the miscarriage as the numbers kept decreasing. I'm not sure if I would feel the same if the cycle just didn't work at all vs. being told you're pregnant and then being told you're not. ☹ It was awful.

It was very devastating.

What Happened – What's Next?

Met with Dr. H a couple of weeks later, 10.26.16. He explained it was nothing I did wrong. It was just not a good embryo. He talked to us about possible PGS if we decided to try again. He also wrote up a new protocol in case we wanted to try again. I had to schedule a semen analysis for Kev. I wanted to see if things had improved or pretty much remained the same. The semen analysis was done on 12.22.16. Results pretty much came back the same, low count, low morphology, same forward progressions, but a bit improved motility. I was wishing the results were significantly better as I'd then try for an IUI vs another fresh cycle. I even had hope of trying on our own. I had a few "late" cycles and symptomatic two-week waits but nothing. That just further solidified the decision to try again!

Anyhow, that was pretty much the gist of the FET cycle.

From Frozen to Fresh

As I mentioned earlier, I've finally decided to go forward with the fresh cycle. I was contemplating waiting for the March cycle to start, but then I realized, why wait, just go for it. So with the onset of the Feb menstrual cycle, I decided to start.

Tuesday — February 21, 2017

I haven't journaled in a couple of weeks. The time is flying; I thought it had only been one week but last entry was 02.10.17. I'm currently on BCP. Started taking them on Tuesday, 02.07.17. Looks like I'll be on them for about 20 days. I haven't really had any side effects except large boobs. They are not sensitive or anything but do seem larger and fuller than normal.

I started Lupron injections on Sunday, 02.19.17. I must tell you that was a mission and a half to get going. I received misdirected info from so many people — namely pharmacy personnel. Margate Specialty Walgreens' originally said I could call a couple days before I needed the Lupron so they could fill the script. That wasn't the case; I found out I had to go through specialty pharmacy, Acredo, not theirs. I then called Acredo and was told Freedom. After having a mini freak-out due to frustration, I finally got script transferred over from Acredo to Freedom and they were able to overnight it to arrive on Saturday, 02.18.17.

It's been two nights since starting the Lupron injections and I think I have slight symptoms, including looser bowels. I also felt hot and sweaty the first night I took it as well. I'm just hoping it gets better or if it doesn't then the time passes quickly.

Unlike with the FET cycle, I am back to icing the injection site before administering it. That has helped a great deal. We're supposed to be going away for the weekend so I plan on taking the ice pack and meds with me. I just hope I don't forget the BCP and injections at home. We took a cruise to Turks and Caicos! It was delightful but yes I was giving myself injections while on the mini-vacation.

Also, I've been in a weird mood. I feel hopeful about the cycle but I am still a bit anxious. I need to call the clinic to find out if they received the labs that my husband and I had done last week. I'm interested to see what the AMH level came back at. Back in August it was 1.53, which is in the good range. Not sure if the number is different if Dr. H will change protocol/meds around a bit. AMH is a hormone level that helps to determine a woman's ovarian reserve. In other words, if the value is in the normal range, then the woman has a good amount of eggs still reserved in her ovaries. This is important for fertility and when doing IVF as it involves follicle stimulation.

Something in me is saying I will not stim for long this cycle. I'm not sure why I feel like this but I do. We'll see. This protocol is now with Gonal-F and Menopur. My previous ones were Follistim and Menopur.

This morning I joined a couple of support groups on Facebook for women who have TACs in place and are undergoing fertility treatments. Looking forward to getting that add'l support from women experiencing similar things.

Monday — February 27, 2017

It's Monday!!! I just returned from a four-day weekend cruise getaway with my hubby. We had an awesome time. I had some things on my mind worrying me but I prayed about it and asked God to allow me to trust him and let him work. Everything worked out, thank God. I said a prayer of thanks and told him I'm sorry for worrying or thinking too much. Both my husband and I got to work at 11 a.m. and 11:30a.m. respectively.

I think it was important to have that alone time to talk about some things and connect together before things take another change in our lives when it comes to having another baby.

My hubby is very excited about going through the process — he's all on board. He was too cute during the trip ensuring I took my meds and did my Lupron injection and kept my medicine cool.

I did join that FB group about IVF and TAC and so far it's been helpful to read and follow other women's stories. It truly is a situation where you are not alone.

We are starting to gear up to start stims on Friday, 03.03.17. The appt is at 7 a.m. Not sure how I'm going to get the boys up and ready so early but it'll get it done — not going to worry about it. I'm hoping all comes back OK with the blood work and ultrasound so I can start with the Menopur and Gonal F. I need to call the Walgreen's Pharmacy to find out if I can use a couple of coupons that I found online. Fingers crossed for that one. It would truly help a great deal.

During our weekend getaway we talked about what to do regarding the transfer — one or two embryos? We are leaning toward only one but the thought of two is still in the very back of our minds. It's just going to be very hard juggling another set of twins. So we'll see what happens when the time comes to actually decide.

I'm really hoping and praying that this cycle works. I do have an overwhelming feeling that it will but still going to take things one day at a time, remain positive and pray. I am also looking forward to an acupuncture treatment scheduled for Wed evening. If I don't have a menstrual cycle, Dr. Duro can do the Mayan abdominal treatment as well.

I took the last BCP on Sunday, 02.26.17. I was excited about that because it marked the end of step one of this journey. I was on them this time for 20 days. Seemed like forever when I first started but now it feels like it actually went by fast. Now, I'm only on the Lupron injections, 10 IU each night. I can actually give myself the injections without icing. My left side doesn't hurt as much — feels kind of numb, actually. Now the right side is totally different. That needle hurts upon it first touching my skin but then it's over once I get it pushed through.

I definitely will have to ice before injecting the other meds, though, because yeah, no.

OK, there's about another hour until I call it a night. Want to get off by 6 so I can see the boys. I haven't seen them since Thursday afternoon before we left for the cruise. It was great hearing from them a couple of hours ago, though, when they came from school ☺.

Thursday March 9, 2017

To say I've been extremely busy is an understatement! Things have been hectic but good, thank God. I am currently on Day 7 of stimulation medications. I feel I am responding extremely well. I'm keeping my fingers crossed things continue to go this way.

On the baseline/stim start appt, last Friday, 03.03.17, I had 15 antral follicles. There were 8 on one side and 7 on the other. My E2 was at 24, nice and low where it should be. My lining was at 4.2. I had just started to bleed as my cycle began a day before, on Thursday 03.02.17.

I am on 75 Menopur and 75 Gonal-F in the morning and the same in the evening. I also take Lupron in the evenings. No more birth control pills, thank goodness. But I started feeling weird when I started the stimulations. However, the night sweats stopped. I did pick up headaches as a new symptom. I think they are worse because of some unfavorable situations at work. Nothing bad, just weird people — hey, you can't please everyone so I'm not going to worry about it anymore!

OK, so as of yesterday, Day 6 of meds, my E2 was 550 and my lining was 6.5mm and I had 13 follicles ranging from 6.6mm (that one showed up from nowhere) to 14.3mm. I needed to purchase meds for Day 8, Friday, so I asked the nurse if I should also get enough for Sat, Day 9, and she said not yet, just order enough to get me through Friday, and depending on my results Friday morning, they'll let me know more. I feel good about that as it means I'm almost ready. I had this overwhelming feeling I'd stim only for 8 days (through Friday, 03.10) so we'll see. I do think I may stim on Saturday to help any additional little ones catch up. That would put my retrieval any day between Sun, 03.12, and

Tues, 03.14. I was hoping for a Sunday retrieval (God's will, of course) as that means I wouldn't have to miss/call off of work. But I'm OK with calling off on Monday vs. Tuesday, 03.14, as that is my boss' birthday so I want to be here for the celebration. Of course we can do it the day after but it's always nice to do so on the day of. ☺

Currently at work and all is going well. I'm feeling very full in my lower belly but not uncomfortable. You can tell things are cooking in there. I did purchase electrolyte water this past weekend at Costco. After much comparing and label reading, I decided to go with the Propel 0 calorie. It is really good! I have also been doing the acupuncture and eating my protein as recommended. That has helped as I am kind of bloated but not in pain, at least not yet. I'm looking forward to picking up my meds tonight. I'll try and leave before 6 so I can head up to Margate Walgreens. I then have to look forward to my appointment in the morning for blood draw, to check E2 and ultrasound, to check follicle growth. I am keeping my fingers crossed and prayers going for good news.

Friday, March 10, 2017

I recently got in to work, a little after 11:30 a.m. I wasn't expecting to be so late, though. The office was very busy today so I had to wait a bit. I was also meeting with the nurse for pre-op, which I was not expecting either. Nurse Beverly went over everything in detail, so it took a while to get through all.

So it doesn't look like I will be triggering tonight. My largest follicles are at 16, so they need another day or so before they're ready. So she explained more than likely I'll have to go back tomorrow morning. I stopped by Walgreen's and ordered/picked up one Menopur and one Gonal-F to get me through Saturday morning. Based on the results of E2 and follicle scan, I'll know if need to buy more. I am really hoping they are ready to go by Saturday. This would mean Monday retrieval. We'll see how it all goes.

I am feeling really sore and bloated in the lower abdomen area. I do feel the crampiness in my ovaries as well. Of course, everything is bearable but definitely sore and uncomfortable. I am also very interested to see how my E2 comes back. They do not want it over 3,000.

My lining showed up at 6.2mm. I asked Nurse Bev about that as on Wed it was 6.5. She did say that is fluctuates sometimes and not to worry about it right now. If I need more support they'll add the estrogen, which I have a prescription for anyway. The reason I was able to know about the 16mm and the lining is that Colleen printed out a follicle scan report and Nurse Bev shared it with me.

It is already 1:30 p.m. and no updated portal message. I am anxiously awaiting that update.

It is now 2:30 p.m. I received the alert of a new portal message a few minutes after 2 p.m. I am to continue on my same dosage for tonight and tmrw morning. Thank goodness I purchased the dose for the morning already. That way I can go straight home tonight. I hope to get some rest/sleep as I have to be up early to get to the clinic at 7:00 a.m. My estrogen is at 1,001 and I have 15 follicles. The leading ones are at 16+, almost 17.

I sent the nurse (Brittany) a message asking if she thinks I'll trigger tonight or Sunday and estimated retrieval date. I also told her I had enough meds to get through tomorrow morning's appt and will wait until the afternoon to see if I need to buy more meds. I am awaiting her response.

I feel a little better about the results today after seeing how they were laid out on the grid. It is much or organized and you get to see how much each follicle has grown in comparison to its last measurement. Continuing to stay positive and hopeful this works for us again and we bring home a healthy baby!

Monday, March 13, 2017

I'm happy to report that all went well over the weekend. I went in for blood work and ultrasound on Saturday and Sunday. On Saturday, E2 was 1996, still had 16 follicles but largest ones were a little over 18. On Sunday, I still had 15 and E2 was 2403 and largest ones were over 21. I received a call on Sunday afternoon that I would be administering the trigger shot Sunday night. So, that is after a full nine days of stimming.

At first I felt kind of bummed as that meant retrieval would be on Tuesday and I'd miss my boss' birthday luncheon, but then I snapped out of it as this is God's will and everything will be fine! The lady on the phone gave me all the instructions and advised they'd also have it up on the portal. I noticed when I checked the portal that they forgot to upload the latest grid based on the Sunday morning appt so I requested they send it. I received it on Monday morning when I asked the receptionist to please get a message to the nurses.

I had blood work this morning at 8:15 — I was late though, arrived at 8:30. Ms. Paula drew blood for hCG, E2, and P4. They mainly want to ensure the trigger shot was done correctly.

My friend, Mary Anne, agreed to give me the shot last night at exactly 10:30 p.m. I didn't feel a thing. The five minutes of ice I applied prior to the shot worked wonders!

I think I am now feeling the effects of the hCG because I am so sleepy sitting here at my desk. Of course nothing goes smoothly all the time. I got to work after11 a.m. as Kason woke up with red puffy eyes so I took him in the pediatrician to be seen. Thank goodness they say it looks to be allergies vs pink eye. So he is home with grandma (thank God for her). Kamden should be home any minute now so I know they will be happy to be reunited. ☺

So, all of that is to say tomorrow is the big day. I am very excited. I also spoke to the anesthesiologist this morning, as well. Their office called me yesterday, yes on Sunday, to get their payment too, LOL. So we are all set.

I sent a message to Dr. Duro as she will not be in after Wednesday this week. She says I can still keep my Wednesday appointment and she will incorporate a pre-transfer treatment as well. I won't see her again until the following Wednesday so I'm going to try and not freak out about not having my second treatment that week. She feels I'm fine and covered and all will be OK. God willing it is!

So now I am thinking about if we're going to have a 3- or 5-day transfer. A 3-day transfer means Friday (another day off of work for both hubby and I this week). A 5-day transfer means Sunday. My first pregnancy was a 5-day. We transferred 2 blasts and only 1 stuck — our precious Angel. Then all 5 remaining embryos did not make it to freeze — they arrested. ☹ Our second pregnancy was a 3-day transfer — we transferred 2 and we now have Kason and Kamden. We had 1 embryo make it to freeze. You just never really know. So, that is also something I am going to try and not worry about because I have no control anyway. God is in control! Until next time!

Wednesday, March 15, 2017

I'm back today with an update. I must say it's very therapeutic for me to write ☺. It's almost 4 p.m. I am back to office after going home to get my boys off of the school bus.

OK, so yesterday was a big day. We arrived at the clinic at 8:30 as scheduled. Check-in was a breeze and they almost immediately took my husband off to give his sample. We first had to verify our identities and sign off on some consents or something. I then went back and changed out of my clothes and into the gown and socks.

My husband came back a little while later. In the meantime, Crystal was the nurse and she was very helpful and nice. She took my vitals and then started the iv. It actually didn't hurt very much — just a little prick and it was in. Granted, she used the same arm I've been getting my blood drawn from and not my hand. I hate hand IVs. Although they are convenient, they hurt like heck.

There was a transfer before mine. They took the first lady in around 9:20ish or maybe it was around 9:30ish. Then it was my turn. I used the restroom and then it was time to go into the OR. Said bye to my hubby and I was off. Dr. Barrioneuvo was doing the retrieval. He always has the nicest and more encouraging words to share with us patients. ☺ I remembered verifying my name and DOB with the nurse lady and then I remembered having to scoot down in the right position in the stirrups. Then I remembered the anesthesiologist almost tripping over something and then he headed back to my head area. I think I then remember/feeling them placing a canula in my nose and that was it. I remember waking up back in the area I started off in. I heard hubby's voice and saw Crystal, I think, but not much else. It took me a while to wake back up. Oh and I remember asking for pain meds and being a bit nauseous.

All of that to say, when I was back fully, I asked about the number of eggs and they told me 16. I was happy with that number. Around 12 noon we were leaving the clinic. Debbie wheeled me downstairs and waited while hubby pulled up the car. We then drove home and I rested for the rest of the day basically. I felt like having scrambled eggs so I asked my mom-in-law, MIL, to make them for me with some wheat toast.

Debbie told me they'd call me between 9 a.m. and noon with a fertilization report. Well I got the call around 7:44 a.m and I thought it was the gate calling for the school bus. Rather, it was the clinic. Debbie said of the 16 eggs, 11 were mature and of the 11, 6 are showing signs of fertilization. I was kind of expecting about 12 mature eggs based on my estrogen — it was at 2,403 when hCG shot was done. So average is 200 per mature follicle. So that was OK. Now I wasn't expecting only 6 fertilizing. I expected more but you just never know. So, I'm happy with the 6 we have so far.

Debbie also said that they'd call us between 8 and 9 a.m. on Friday to let me know if we need to go in for the transfer on Friday. She explained that if we have a couple that are ahead more than the rest then they would want to transfer them back to me rather than wait. If all show signs of progressing, then they'd wait and perform a 5-day transfer on Sunday.

I am praying all goes well accordingly to God's will. He has showed me time and time again that I need not worry but somehow I tend to do so. I guess I am just nervous and want everything to go well. My family and I are no better than anyone else so I try to stay humble and grateful at the same time through all of our feats. I am praying for a 5-day transfer and I'm just not sure about how the 6 will do. So in the meantime I will be sending positive vibes and prayers for our 6 babies to grow, grow, grow and be healthy. It's weird too because I also worried about having too many and having to make the decision after they've been frozen of what to do with them :/ But God sees and knows everything.

I sent a message to hubby about the fertilization report and he called back wanting me to explain it a bit more to him. He's now worried and thinking about if we should transfer 1 or 2. He feels that if they are 3-day then maybe 2 would optimize the chances but not sure about how they'll do waiting until 5 days. In the meantime, we will take things one day at a time. I have acupuncture today at 6 so I'm looking forward to that treatment. Dr. Duro will not be in the rest of the week so this treatment will also serve as a pre-transfer treatment as well. I am keeping my fingers crossed and praying for everything.

By the way, hubby still doesn't want me to say anything to anyone so only one of my closest friends knows. He wants us to keep this to ourselves so we can take it all in and decide when the time is right to share the, prayerfully, good news.

Tuesday, March 21, 2017 — 2dp5dt

Since my last update last week, there have been some uneventful and some very eventful days! Thursday, 03.16.17, was a normal day for me. I stayed and worked until about 7:30pm because I missed Tuesday as I was out sick. In the meantime, we were anxiously awaiting the call from the clinic regarding how the embryos were doing on day 3. That call would determine if I'd go in on Friday for the transfer, day 3, or I'd go in on Sunday, day 5.

Friday, 03.17.17, rolled around and I was nervously awaiting the phone call. My husband went off to work as usual. We planned to have my oldest son Rich drive me there and then hubby would take a break and come to pick me up. When I spoke to Mrs. Debbie on Wednesday, she said they would call on Friday between 8 and 9 a.m. Well I wasn't sure if I should go to work or wait but it was indeed nerve-wracking. We prayed day and night for the embryos to make it to blastocyst stage. My good friend and her mom were praying for us as well. ☺ Well, I got the call at like 8:49 a.m. and it was Crystal. She said she had good news and that we would go for the 5-day transfer on Sunday. I asked her if we still had the 6 embryos from Wednesday and she said yes! I was shocked and floored and very grateful at the same time. God was hearing us loud and clear. We prayed for his will be done so we can end up with a successful full-term pregnancy. Even though I wouldn't have minded a 3-day transfer, as my twin boys were 3-day transfers, we just really wanted to know we had enough strong babies to try and go to 5-day. I asked about the quality and she explained that they didn't really say much, but we're good for Sunday.

So, then a few minutes later as I'm prepping to go to work the phone rings. I looked and saw the clinic was calling me back. I for a short minutes started to panic but figured it is what it is. I thought they were calling to say they made a mistake and I was to come in that day. Well, it was Mrs. Debbie. She called to reassure me and to see how I am as she knows how nervous I was when I called her back a couple days later. I thought that was the sweetest thing ever! When I called her I was saying I thought we didn't do well this cycle to have only 11 of 16 mature and only 6 or 11 fertilized. She said we did well and no one there thought we did anything wrong. Only one work day for me. She also explained that she understands our fear as we dedicate time money and energy in this whole process so it's only normal for us to want a great outcome. So she called and said she noticed that Crystal had called me already but she wanted to speak with me herself as well. She said, "See? Everything is fine and will be OK and it worked out." ☺ I asked about the quality and she explained that we still had 6 but 5 were perfect and the other one just slightly behind but not bad by any means. I am extremely happy. I called Kev to give him the news and he was ecstatic as well! I went on to have a normal Friday.

Oh, Debbie also explained that she had two patients on Thursday and one of them had 4 embryos and when they checked on Day 3 only 1 was ahead so they called her in to do a 3-day transfer. The other patient had 5 embryos and 3 were ahead so they called her and told her they were aiming for a 5-day transfer. So you see how it's kind of like a numbers game to some extent.

Saturday, March 18, 2017 — I went on to have a good, busy day. I was up early and went to Sawgrass Mall to shop for my nephew, Narvens' 5th bday gift. He wanted light-up shoes from sketchers. It was also Jahsai's 18th bday so I picked up a gift card for him. I also re-upped on my skin/face care items from Body shop. Oh and I purchased 3 parfums — I love them, LOL. I then went home, picked up the boys, and took them to the birthday party. We were there for a while. After a few hours, I left them at my brother's house and went to work at my office for a few hrs. I then went to Publix and Dollar Tree, mainly to buy the pineapple and brazil nuts. I found the last pineapple in the store. Also, there were no pkgs of brazil nuts but I got a mixture that had some in there so I bought two of those. I then went back to pick up the boys, sat around and played some games with my older nieces and nephew, and then went home. I was tired, LOL — it was a long day.

Sunday, March 19, 2017 — Embryo Transfer Day — I decided to go to 7:30 a.m. Mass on Sunday. I don't like to miss church. We had to be at the clinic at 9:00 a.m. Mass was great, as usual. I then got ready, and hubby and I left.

Of course there was some unforeseen incident on the turnpike. It looked like a car fire. But thank goodness it cleared up soon after we got on. Like I predicted, we got to the clinic at 9:15 a.m. There were only three of us patients there, two retrievals and me a transfer.

The lab picked the two best embryos for us to transfer. The nurse, Melody, went to ask because we hadn't decided if we were doing one or two. She came back and explained that they chose two because there was no indication on our paperwork and for our age, two is the most they'd do with this good quality. I asked if we could talk to Dr. Barrionuevo about it. He said he agreed we should do only the one given our history. So the lab updated the report and the nurse brought us the picture of the embryo — it looked beautiful! Hubby and I shot a couple of selfies with the baby. ☺ I then took the Valium, drank another cup of water. Another nurse came with an ultrasound machine to see how full my bladder was. She said they like it to be full but not uncomfortable. They like to see 200ml, well mine was filled at 327ml, smh.

We walked in to the o/r after both my husband and I changed into the gowns. I didn't start feeling the effects of the valium as soon as I normally do. But I was still relaxed, nonetheless. That darned speculum is always uncomfortable, but once we bypassed that I didn't really feel much else. Dr. B gave us his faith-filled speech, which I love. The embryologist, Ryan, came by to verify my name and date of birth. Dr. B was also checking the uterus cavity and he said what a beautiful lining. I asked how thick is it and he measured and said 11.1mm. I was blown away! I've never had a lining that thick, I don't think. Normally during stims I get to 7.3 and then 6.7 and I think I was at 6.5 before I stopped stims this last go round. During my last FET, I think it was at 6.3 and Doc H put me on vaginal Estrace and during my consult after the early miscarriage he said it had gotten up to 10mm for transfer. I remember that I forgot to ask Dr. B how much the lining was as the Valium had already kicked in and I was not all there.

Anyway, I was very happy to hear about the 11.1mm lining. That means it's nice and cushy in there for the little baby. ☺

Then they positioned the catheter, and they called for the embryo. It was brought out and placed inside. Dr. B asked me to look at the screen and I'll see when/where it's deposited. It was beautiful and placed perfectly. I then received a print of the transfer pic. Dr. B made sure hubby and I gave each other a nice kiss right before the transfer and another one right after — it was very sweet of them.

I was then told to lie there for about a minute and then slide to the bottom of the table. I then stood up, walked out, and went to the original area where we were waiting. The nurse instructed me to go to the restroom and place the Crinone in and urinate. I did then go back and changed into my clothes. They needed to go and check something so while they were away I just rested there for another 15–20 minutes or so. They then came back and I think we signed some docs, don't really remember, then we got the OK to go! They explained the final embryo report would be ready on Tuesday and I'd hear back from them then to find out how many made it to freeze. I asked will normally they call the next day. She explained that they do freeze on the next day but they'll notify on the day the final report was ready. The ride home was nice, too. We were home in no time. I immediately got home and went upstairs to my room and rested.

That was pretty much the rest of my Sunday. I didn't really feel much outside of being a bit tired. I went and had dinner with hubby downstairs while the boys were still napping around after 4:30ish.

I then got back in to bed. The boys came up for bed and thank goodness they didn't really give me a hard time to fall asleep, so I didn't do too much moving to get them settled. I then tried to stay up and watch TV or YouTube but I was done and tired. I turned everything off, said a prayer, and went to bed.

Monday, March 20, 2017 — 1dp5dt — I got up and Rich helped me get the boys ready for school. That was pretty uneventful. I tried not to lift them too much. Once they were off, I decided to just take a shower because I didn't want to place a new Crinone in and it was all weird down there, LOL. I wanted to start with a clean slate!

After my shower I had breakfast, took my vitamins, ate my pineapple, nuts, etc. I tried to watch TV but wasn't really paying much attention to it. I then wanted to watch Wendy, but it was then cut off for a live broadcast of something about Trump and the Russian influence and wiretapping allegations. I then stopped fighting my sleep and was knocked out. I asked my husband to call and wake me at 12:30 but that didn't happen. I jumped up and it was already 1:00 p.m. So I arrived at work around 1:30 p.m.

The rest of the day was good. I still wasn't feeling much discomfort just slight pinches and twinges. Oh, I forgot to mention, in the morning I felt like I had to go #2 and it was kind of hard. I had been taking Colace since Sat as I hadn't had a BM since egg retrieval on Tuesday. The anesthesia always does a number on my bowels and slows things down. So I finally had the urge to go, but I tried not to strain. I got a bit paranoid and started Googling but all was fine.

While at work, I got a phone call from the clinic. It was Nurse Debbie. ☺ She was calling to tell me that we had three embryos that made it to freeze. There was someone in my office, so I couldn't be as enthused as I wanted to be but I was happy! She was like you see — you did great — isn't that wonderful, everything worked out. She's really a sweetheart. Really helps patients be at ease. I asked about the quality and she said well they have to meet certain criteria to even freeze and the three are the same grade as the one we transferred back so I was very excited about that.

Still the rest of the day was good. Haven't really been feeling much of anything, I have been very gassy since the day of transfer. OMG, it smells so bad too, my poor hubby. The other thing is that I seem to be comfy only on my back to sleep. I hate sleeping on my back, but for the past two days, it's been the best position.

While I sit at my desk and type this — **Tuesday, March 21, 2017** — I feel gassy, and just felt a little sharp twinge on my left side of the uterus. It was hard for me to eat my breakfast this morning too. That was very odd. I didn't really have an appetite or taste for the food — and I LOVE my breakfast. I ate it because I knew I had to. I remember reading somewhere it's best to eat the pineapple core on an empty stomach so that's what I did. Maybe that's why the food wasn't as appetizing to me. Once I finished my food, I had an 8 oz. bottle of water and maybe an hr later I had all my vitamins and other meds (prenatal, vit d, dhea, omega fatty acid, Estrace, Colace).

For some reason, I'm looking forward to having the implantation bleeding due to the thick lining, but we'll see. My boobs are heavier, but my nipples although aren't as sore anymore; they are a bit sensitive and the areola was ashy/scaly this morning. As I typed this I felt a slight stinging sensation come down in the left breast/nipple. OK, until next time!

Ok, I'm back 2:04 p.m. I realized when putting my lipstick on this morning that my lips seemed kind of chapped/dry. I didn't think much of it figured; well, I should have put on some Chapstick upstairs. Then I thought well that's weird because the lipstick I was applying is very creamy and that consistency lasts all day pretty much and even when it comes off, my lips are still moisturized. I drink a lot of water daily so this was weird.

Well, fast forward to mid-day and I ran my tongue across my lips and they were chapped, like chapped. Not even rubbing them together helped break up the dryness. I could literally peel the skin off in between the cracked lipstick.

So I went to the oracle, Google, thinking nothing would result but of course there were tons of experiences by other women in which chapped lips were a sign of early pregnancy for them. One post I read said a doc mentioned that the baby sucks all the moisture, which is why some women are very thirsty, have dry skin, dry eyes, dry lips, etc.

OK, we'll see by next week if this holds true. ☺ And my goodness, the GAS! Awful, still. Thinking we want to test Saturday morning as that will be 6 days post-transfer. I'm so anxious to do it though.

Wednesday, March 22, 2017 — 3dp5dt

Not much to report today but wanted to come on and journal. I am now 3dp5dt. I don't really feel much but some slight twinges or cramps but they don't last long at all and don't really hurt much either. I did have some sharp pains in the vaginal area but they didn't last long, either. I do feel very tired and out of breath after walking, especially up and down the stairs at home. My boobs do not hurt, but they are full and the nipples are dark and pronounced. They are sensitive to the touch only a bit and only at certain times, not constant.

I am trying to be positive about the whole thing. I didn't feel like having my normal waffles and peanut butter for breakfast this morning. I was up very early, before my alarm. So I got the kids ready for school and hung out with them downstairs until the bus came. I then took the time to boil two eggs and have my pineapple. I ate the eggs on my way to work and had a bottle of water.

I then had my green drink around 11:30 a.m. and ate the nut mixture I had left. For some reason I'm still waiting and checking for implantation spotting or bleeding. I don't feel anything else major going on but I just have this strong sense that I am pregnant. My husband called to check on me because I have one of his chickens in me, smh. ☺

I have acupuncture later this evening and am looking forward to that. I can't wait to share the updates with Dr. Duro. I am going to make a call to Mrs. Debbie to ask about how they freeze the embryos — separately or together. I'll also ask her about the whole assisted hatching and how that plays in to the final bill, too.

The funny thing is this cycle feels familiar in that it's mimicking my first fresh cycle. I really didn't feel much until I had 2–3 days of implantation bleeding. The 3rd day I had a big appetite and lower back pain and slight spotting. I thought for sure my cycle was coming. But I don't remember feeling anything really until 6dp5dt, which was four days before my beta. Granted, back then I had never been pregnant before so I didn't know any better. I was just afraid. I am saying my prayers and trying to stay busy with work, etc., as to minimize my time to have weird thoughts. We're just really wishing everything works out. God doesn't want us to worry, so I really try not to.

OK, so I called Debbie. She explained in the recent past they used to do two embryos to a vial. She also mentioned the latest practice has been to store them individually as they have been doing more and more single embryo transfers so she wants to say they are individually frozen right now but she's not totally for sure as she's not working in the lab.

I also asked about the assisted hatching. She gave me Mandee's number in financial to ask her as it may depend on what package I had as there are different ones offered. She did explain that they typically do it on patients over 40 for fresh cycles and for all cryo (FET) cycles. I called and left a message for Mandee. So I'll ask her if that amount will be deducted from my final bill as we did not do it.

Thursday, March 23, 2017 — 4dp5dt

I didn't get a chance to update after my call to Mandee. She explained that AH is included in the price given we do or don't do it. We went over some other stuff, too. That reminds me, I need to contact BCBSIL as they did not pay for a visit back in 10.26.16, or post-miscarriage doc visit, so that balance was applied against my loan. So once I go to do the blood test, I'll have to pay a balance of about $76.

OK so the rest of the day, yesterday, 03.22.17, was weird. I was very hungry and I had this dull crampy sensation on the right side of my uterus. Then I went to stand up from my desk and got this sharp pain that ran from the top of by belly button down to the bottom part of my uterus. It was as if someone took a knife and sliced right through in that straight line. It was awful. I had to slowly move while it went away. It kind of lasted for a minute or so. Then the sharp pain was gone but behind my belly button area was still a bit achy.

Then as the day progressed, I was ready to go home. I had acupuncture and was happy to go as I hadn't seen Dr. FD for a week. The treatment was a good one. I was able to update her on everything that transpired during the past week. She was excited and said I responded extremely well and that I had the ovaries of a 20-yr-old. ☺ She felt my pulse nice and strong as well.

Driving home was a chore though. I was ready to get there asap. I felt nice and relaxed after the treatment but felt a little icky, too; I needed to rest. I got home, took a shower, and got in bed. I then stated to feel a dull cramp that was steady on my right side. If I lay in a particular position, I wouldn't feel much, but when I got up to walk to the bathroom or something I definitely felt it. Then I was hungry. I didn't want to eat cereal, but my hubby didn't look like he was in the mood to go anywhere — he had already fallen asleep — so I just had the last bit of milk with the cereal. I felt better afterward and had a lot of gas/burps. I sat up for a few minutes and then turned everything off. I was still on my phone following videos of a couple I found but then went to sleep.

I felt a bit weird too because I was having dreams that I felt weren't really dreams but felt more like I was awake. Anyway, I got up this morning, 03.23.17, and said I'm going to take a test. I said well since it's only been 3 days (surely I was confused because it was 4 days past transfer) I'll just do it to ensure trigger is out — which I knew it should've been out already — and if it came back negative I'll know for sure that the weekend results would be good. So it was 6:55 a.m. and I must've urinated in a cup and dropped the droplets onto the test window around 6:56 a.m.

It was taking a while — or at least longer than I wanted to wait, LOL — and dropped more urine in. I finished up and washed the cup and went on about my business because by the time I finished peeing, the sample had gone through the window completely and it looked to me like there was nothing there. So I got the boys up and proceeded to get them ready for school.

I then came back up and started to make my bed and was feeling bad saying oh my goodness I know it's early but what if it didn't work and all this crazy stuff. Then suddenly as I was making my husband's side I said no, why wouldn't it work, everything was going well outside the uterus and the embryo did what it was supposed to do so why wouldn't it do so back inside. I'm going to be confident and know that God heard of dreams and he will provide for us and that was that.

So I proceeded to take out my brush to brush my teeth and then go shower then I said well let me move this test and put it away. It had been a good 30 minutes or so by now. I looked at it and by darned there seemed to be a line! + So I walked around with it to see if it was for real. I then dropped to my knees, saying thank you, God. I got nervous, LOL. Then I started taking pictures, LOL. My hands and feet got really sweaty during the whole process.

I then took my shower and while doing so was talking to God, LOL. ☺ We had a nice conversation about me continuing to learn not to worry and knowing he'll take care of me because that's what he promised. I then repeated my prayers for my husband too. I haven't told my hubby yet. I guess I'm waiting to ensure the weekend test gets darker and then show him the one I took this morning. I don't know yet though what I'll do.

I got ready for work and stopped at Dunkin Donuts for a bagel as we were out at home. Of course I forgot the apple juice. So I called a friend and her hubby dropped off orange juice for me. In the meantime, I had my last day of pineapple on an empty stomach and then my breakfast and then my vitamins.

I've since been OK, just dull cramps and yawning a lot at my desk as I work. Hopefully, I can have lunch in another hour before 3 p.m. I like to wait for my boss. ☺ We'll see how long that'll last though, LOL.

I'm so excited and because I promised not to worry, I won't. Just going to take things one day at a time and know that since the little baby implanted, based on hCG in urine, then he/she will continue to grow and develop.

I did a Google search to find out the sensitivity of the HPT test I used this morning. It was called First Signal and I bought it from the $Tree. I found that it picks up a level of at least 25 miu. So that's definitely a good sign. With the FET miscarriage, my hCG beta came back at 10 so.

I am very excited and just trying to take things one day at a time and while praying for continued success. Until next time.

<u>Friday, March 24, 2017 — 5dp5dt</u>

Last night was definitely an ordeal for me. Ok, so I got home a little after 7 p.m. as I left the office late. The rest of the day was OK symptom-wise. I felt hungry and a bit more out of breath. I felt some moisture down there too. I thought it was implantation spotting but nothing. I still had a bout with gas as well. I got home and was out of breath as I explained a story to my husband of what happened at work. I then took my shower and got into bed. I was having constant little cramping sensations. It was not unbearable but definitely pronounced. Also I had trapped gas in my back as it felt like it was making its way up my spine. I felt a bit scared for a moment and just tried not to breathe too hard or move too fast until it moved on out.

When it was actually time to fall asleep I had a hard time doing so. I kind of know I'm pregnant, too, because I'm the most comfortable sleeping on my back and that's a big no-no for me. Well, I also had a bad bout of itching. Every part of my body itched. It was uncomfortable. My head, arms, back, eyes, everything was itchy. I also had a bout of discomfort and realized my left leg was achy and hurt from the lower hip/upper thigh part all the way down to my feet. I then looked at my phone. It was like 11:10 p.m. and I had been feeling the pain for about 10 minutes. I think it finally went away maybe close to 11:30 p.m. It was very achy and almost charley horse/cramp-like. Thank goodness it stopped, though. I do remember getting leg cramps during other early pregnancy waits as well. So that was also a good sign to me.

Oh, I forgot to mention I was extremely hungry, too. My husband offered to go and get something for me, but I didn't want him to leave again so I just bore with it and told him I'd just have a large breakfast. I felt even more hungry because I couldn't sleep. I prayed I would go down and finally I did — not sure what time it was, though.

I was up early again around the time of my husband's wake up alarm. I felt OK. I was hungry and felt like I had a hole under my breastbone. I drank water and it kind of hurt a bit, too, but felt I needed it because I was thirsty.

I still haven't told my husband that I took the HPT yesterday. We talked about taking one tomorrow, Saturday morning, instead of waiting until Sunday. I'm just taking things one day at a time and it's funny because I don't worry anymore. I have this overwhelming sense of calm. I think it's because I saw the + so now I'm not second guessing everything. ☺ I'm just keeping the faith that all will continue to work out.

I had a nasty incident this morning that I almost forgot to mention. After I had the sips of water I felt I needed to go, so I did #2.

I then brushed my teeth and showered. While drying myself off, I felt like I had to pass gas. Well I was trying to pass gas and bam it was loose #2 instead. I was shocked because I normally always know the difference between gas and that, LOL. Well, I was sadly mistaken. So I went to the toilet and finished my business. It was definitely a lot of #2. I am not sure where all that came from because when I went before my shower it was nice and solid. So I immediately thought, "OK, there's another sign." I remember having this for other cycles as well. I then remember Lourdes saying she knew something was weird because she kept pooping a lot when she got pregnant with Olivia.

So, it's a little after 11 a.m. now. I'm going to continue my work day. I did get a call back from Mandee, and she explained that the office tried to rebill the 10.26.16 visit back in Jan 2017 and it also got denied. They sent the bill again with the same code so they'll use another code and if it gets paid, they'll reimburse me the $230. It can take 4–6 weeks, though.

I am looking forward to the weekend although it's a busy one. I have to get my hair relaxed, acupuncture, and then attend a women's conference with my friend Maria. I'm hoping to go to the grocery store tonight with my husband and the boys since I won't have time to do it tomorrow. When I come home from the conference, I can already see my bed in my head, LOL.

Monday, March 27, 2017 — 8dp5dt

Sigh! Well I'm not sure how I'm doing today as so much has happened over the past couple of days, this past weekend. I'm feeling a little bit down if I am honest but yet I'm also feeling hopefully still. I'm trying not to act too sad either as I have blessed with a lot and I don't want to seem ungrateful.

On Friday when I got off of work, I got home to relieve Rich. I then spent some time with Kamden as Kason had fallen asleep after his bath. I then went to lie down as I waited for my husband to get home. The plan was for us to go to the grocery stores and get that out of the way since I had a busy Saturday. So we went to Costco and Walmart. Nothing much happened except for feeling tired and some sharp quick pains in my uterus area. We made it home and were done with everything close to 9 p.m. I'm not sure what else happened, but I think I was hungry and had some cereal so we didn't have to leave the house again and that was that.

On the next day, **Saturday — 6dp5dt,** I was up early as I had a hair appointment at 8:30. I made some breakfast and ate it in the car on my way to the appt. After the hair appointment I had acupuncture at noon so I made it to that appt about 10 minutes early. After acupuncture, I ran an errand to ensure the a/c guy was paid. Something happened and they needed to clean and flush out the system. I was home for a quick minute and then left again as I needed to attend a women's conference Maria invited me to for St. Stephen AME church. The conference was at Shula's Hotel in Miami Lakes.

I am really happy I was able to attend, although I was a little late. I arrived just as the ladies were concluding lunch. It was indeed very enlightening and empowering. Truly amazing to see God working in our midst.

Then I called to see if Grandma, my MIL, was ready to be picked up, so I headed down south to Nezie's house to pick her up. I then stopped at a restaurant to buy food for the boys and then McDonald's for myself. We finally got back home around 7 p.m. Needless to say, I was exhausted and tired. I then remember getting ready for bed.

I forgot to mention that I took an HPT early in the morning before I left for my hair appt. I used the $tree test and it did come back + again but still faint. I still felt hopeful. I then started to feel worried because I thought it'd be darker than it was on Thursday since it had been two days later. While at the salon I sent a text to my friend and explained and she said not to worry as just as the docs, and everyone says and knows, it's in God's hands now. That made me feel a bit better. I still hadn't told my husband that I took the first and now second test.

Before getting ready for bed, I asked hubby to come with me to buy a real test so that I would know for sure instead of messing around with the $tree in case it wasn't clear. We rode to CVS and bought a First Response. I told him I'd take it Sunday morning and I didn't want him to tell me what it said.

The next day, Sunday — 7dp5dt — I got up and took the FRER and then got back into bed. Long story short, I couldn't tell what my husband was thinking. I asked him to let me see the test after he said aloud it was negative (-). I thought he was joking. I'm learning to not let him talk me in to these things because it just gets you down and it's hard to get back out of it after seeing a result you weren't expecting. So I looked and it was in fact negative, not even the slightest faint line. I felt bad but still not too worried as I figured it was just too early as I know some people test + at 9dp5dt. I promised myself I would not test anymore and wait until the official test on Wednesday.

Needless to say, we were still a bit silent and not sure how to feel. I then got up and ready for church. The service was great, as usual. I then went home, ate breakfast, took my vitamins and got in to bed. I took a great nap for about three hours. I had some twinges and cramps, etc., as well that lasted well into the rest of the day and overnight. Some of them were sharp, too. I just don't know.

I am just trying to remain hopeful. I must say though that it was funny to hear my husband say that when we do it again he's transferring two, and we'll take our chances. That makes me feel better to know that he's at least on board to try again. I really hope we don't need to but at least we have embryos just in case.

Monday, March 27, 2017 – 8dp5dt

I took the time out of my morning to write this up. I am now going to continue with the rest of my day and try not to think about things too much. God's got me — I just know he does! I'm just praying this desire we have is in line with his timing and plans for us.

It's now a little after 2 p.m. I am feeling a lot better mood-wise. I said my prayers during a walk break outside. I have also been having some sharp cramps and twinges this morning as well but I am not going to read too much into them. I am also still very thirsty but trying to spread my water bottles.

I spoke with my friend about everything and that is when I finally shed some tears. I haven't since this whole up and down roller coaster craziness. I have to keep remembering that there is nothing we can do now except pray.

<u>Tuesday — March 28, 2017 — 9dp5dt</u>

I woke up to some weird/scary dreams this morning. In order to fall back asleep, I put my rosary under my belly and didn't get up again until Rich knocked on the door. It was 4 minutes past 7 at that time. I started feeling a little down again this morning. I've been saying my prayers and trying to remain calm and positive.

I felt a bit of a lower dull back ache this morning when getting the kids ready for school. I remember feeling the same way right before being pregnant with Angel. I don't remember it too much with the boys but I'm sure it was the same as with the boys I remember my stomach gurgling and thinking my period was coming any minutes as I also felt moisture down there too. I don't feel any moisture and my bowel movement was normal this morning not runny. There wasn't much but it was more solid.

My boobs are feeling the same as before both pregnancies too. They are not overly sensitive or too swollen. They are definitely plump and the nipples have dry spots on them that I can actually peel off. However, they are not extremely sensitive to the touch.

I got a little bit of hope last night as I watched a YouTube video of a lady "forgot the tots" where she tested with a faint positive at 5dp5dt and then negative, no line at all, at 6dp5dt. Then she dropped the sample in the sink when she went to test at

7dp5dt. So she said it must've meant she wasn't supposed to test and left it alone. She had beta done at 9dp5dt and it came back at 26. The nurse was not optimistic at all and told her to come back 4 days later. That beta came back at over 100, I want to say like 160. Then she went back two days later and it was at 352 or something and then two days after that it was 670. So they scheduled her ultrasound and all of that to say she is doing OK and delivered a healthy baby girl. I think at her first u/s at 8 weeks the baby was three days behind. Then at the 12-week u/s the baby caught up. So she was someone who had late implantation maybe or just a slow grower. I am hoping that is the case with me when I go for beta tmrw, that I am indeed pregnant just took a little longer to show up. I am sooooo anxious yet will continue to pray. Last night I felt some dull cramps and some sharp twinges in the belly button area and in the uterine area. They don't last long but they are there.

The lady also said that she didn't feel any cramps or anything mainly until about 7dp5dt. I also had more cramping that started Sunday, 7dp5dt. I just don't know. At least there is only one more day to wait as I go in tomorrow morning to get the blood drawn.

I forgot my morning dose of vitamins at home. I did remember the Crinone, so that's good. I am not too worried, though, but I will go home for a quick moment to take them at noon or so. I really don't want to be without the estrogen/Estrace.

It's about 11:18 a.m. I am feeling a dull constant back ache along with a dull lower uterine cramping sensation. It's a feeling like I need to put a heating bad on my belly and back — weird to explain. Then I got a slight bout of nausea — very weird. Now it's turning into like a weird sensation like I have to use the restroom. I just passed gas and feel a little relief. I'm so afraid and anxious. I'm continuing to pray for the best.

The rest of the day just kind of flew by. I was hungry a little earlier than usual so I had lunch closer to 1 p.m. I pretty much felt the same symptoms wise, kind of fast breathing, hungry, thirsty, gassy, etc. I don't really remember many cramps that stood out but I definitely still had them. Also my boobs felt like they were filling up on and off. That was weird.

I got home a little bit after 7 p.m. I spent time with the boys and couldn't wait to put them to sleep so I could eat my cereal, smh. I did have this weird sore sensation in my uterus. It kind of felt like it was lagging behind when I went to turn or get out of bed. That was weird. My lower to mid/lower back was a bit uncomfortable and I had more stomach gurgling.

I eventually prayed and then went to sleep.

Wednesday, March 29, 2017 — 10dp5dt

I woke up in the middle of the night and it was only 1 a.m. So I said more prayers and eventually fell asleep again. I was then up and watched my husband prep for work. I got up minutes after 6:30 a.m. and got myself ready for the day. I was able to leave the house about the same time as the boys when they got on the bus this morning.

I arrived at the clinic and signed in. The front desk called me up and she asked why I was there. So obviously someone forgot to key in my beta appt, I presume. I told her and she said, "OK I'll put your chart up and good luck!" I smiled and said, "Thank you." The clinic was very busy.

Paula didn't call me until maybe what feels like 15–20 minutes later. As she went to draw the blood, nothing would come out so she had to move the needle around. It didn't hurt but it felt weird. Then eventually it started to pour out and then slowed down, smh. I'm not sure what those two occurrences were about but glad it's over and I'll chalk it up to, well, sometimes things happen, we're human ☺. I then asked her how long the wait was for the nurse and she said she didn't know but she'd call one for me as both Beverly and Jacki were in. I didn't even sit down for a quick minute and Nurse Brittany called me. I asked about how long do I have to wait in case I want to do an FET. She explained not long at all and that as long as a woman gets a period you can do the FET. I asked if I'd have to be on BCP and she said not necessarily as it depends on what the patient may want and what the doc's schedule would be in case they need to time the transfer for a specific timeframe, etc.

I was then on my way. She wished me luck and I got a bit emotional wishing that I don't need the FET right now or at all because of a fail. She wished me the same thing and said that she'd call me as soon as the number comes in, but the Dr. H would also call. She reminded me it's very busy today and I said, "Yes I know, LOL," so the call would probably be in the afternoon. I've been praying and praying and crossing everything.

I'm now going to try and work until the time comes when the phone rings. I find being busy helps me not think about it as much.

Fresh Cycle Was a Bust – Going to Try Something New

Friday, March 31, 2017

So I am finally able to come back to finalize my journaling for this cycle. I got the call at about 11:21 a.m. from Dr. Hoffman. Just based on the sound of his voice, I knew it wasn't promising news. He said, "the beta came back negative Mar, I'm sorry." I was OK with it for the most part. He then went on and suggested a diagnostic procedure called the (ERA) Endometrial Receptivity Array. It's a biopsy in which they take a bit of the endometrial lining on the day of (supposed) transfer and send it for testing to see if it was indeed "receptive" and ready for the transferred embryo. The results may come back pre-receptive which means the transfer should have been later or post-receptive which means the transfer should've happened earlier. He explains there are certain RNA genes that must be present in the lining for implantation to happen and the test checks to see if the genes that need to be there are actually there. He said it'll be just prepping for a FET cycle, but instead of transferring the embryo, they take a biopsy of the lining and send it off for testing. He then answered a couple more questions that I had. I asked about the cost and he said it may be about $650 or so with the FET medications, but it's worth it. He then explained that Nurse Jacki would call me and we would take it from there. I was also to stop my medications, wait for a period.

I was then looking into ways to see if insurance would pay for it since it's a diagnostic test and insurance doesn't cover infertility. So in speaking with the insurance company on Thursday afternoon, she tried to look up the procedure for me to find a code but it kept coming back as infertility. So, Mandee said I could call and ask the nurses what diagnosis and procedure code they'd use so that I can see if my insurance would cover.

I plan on calling in to the office today because my cycle came last night. I started spotting last night and when I woke up to use the restroom this morning, I had a red flow on the liner.

Although I started my cycle, I am not sure if I can start the process now to get things rolling for the ERA biopsy cycle. I'm still thinking about all the finances involved in this stuff, but I am also trying not to worry about it because it will all work out, it just has to. Some people do it and follow their dreams on much less so I'll continue to pray about it.

I called the office and spoke to Nurse Beverly. She said doc said I could either do the ERA cycle or just go right into another FET cycle. She explained what needed to be done with the ERA biopsy cycle. I decided to go through with the biopsy cycle as I feel it will increase our chances of a subsequent medicated cycle. I will continue to pray about it.

The nurse further explained that I have to do the same protocol for the ERA cycle as the FET cycle. Then she said that they really want to do BCPs because if after the biopsy the results aren't back yet and I get a period, meaning I'm ready to start the FET, they'll have to cancel the cycle. Doing the BCPs help control what happens in the timing after the ERA. So if I get my period, even if results aren't back, I'll be on BCPs so then it's OK to time out the FET transfer.

So, all in all, I go in on Monday, 04.03.17, at 8:15 a.m. for blood work and ultra sound. I'll then see a nurse so I can start BCPs that night. She is also going to send my script to both Freedom and Walgreen's specialty to see how much the prices come back at so I can compare. As much as I wanted to jump right into things because I want to be pregnant already, ☹ I figure I have no choice but to wait and it will be a good thing as I'll be able to figure things out regarding paying for visits, medications, etc.

Thursday, April 13, 2017

It's been a long day. My husband and I were off yesterday. We spent the day with the boys for spring break. We weren't able to take the entire week off but figured we should at least take one day. We had a great time. Being with the boys really help me to not dwell on anything else. ☺ It's such a blessing to have them!

My Rx delivery came on Tuesday, 04.11, from Freedom Pharmacy. It was the Lupron. I am supposed to start on Friday, April 14, 2017. I had to leave right after this because my husband called as something was going on with his car.

Friday, April 14, 2017

It's Good Friday! I'm feeling a bit overwhelmed but it has seemed to have gotten better as the day progressed. I started taking the Lupron this morning. I am also still on bcp. I only have one more week of the BCP as I take the last pill on Fri, 04.21. Ugh, I hate how I feel when I'm on those pills. I know it's necessary.

I had a great day with the boys a couple days ago. I also went home for lunch to drop off plantains and got to see them. ☺ Kason was asleep and Kam was up and at it, as usual. I'm starting to have this feeling of not being afraid to do more and be there more for them. It's really weird and I'm not sure I am explaining it well. I am really enjoying being with them as they are much older and we can actually have conversations and enjoy experiences together. I took them for a walk with me last night and they really enjoyed it. On Wednesday when I was off, I had a fun time running around with them at the water park and then Chuck E. Cheese. I wasn't tired at all. I was actually looking forward to just being in the hectic busy moments with them.

I am really praying that the next FET cycle works for us. I have to get over the whole idea of being older when I have the baby. I think everything happens for a reason and God made it so the boys would be a bit more independent and able to be themselves before he gave us another baby to handle. Although I was and am saddened by the loss back in Oct and the failed IVF fresh cycle last month, I do believe God is looking out for us.

I also like being busy with work, birthdays, the boys, etc., because it helps take my mind off of thinking about the cycle and the upcoming biopsy. I just pray all comes back in a way that will allow us to maximize our chances for success in the next few months. During this Easter season, I just can't help but feel that God got us and He will work it all out for us, as he always does. ☺ God is in control!

Time to do the ERA - The Transfer

May/June 2017

We did the ERA! We followed all of the same steps as if it were an FET. I remember being a bit apprehensive thinking about how the biopsy would be, pain-wise. I have to say it wasn't that bad. Dr. Hoffman wanted to make sure he got enough of a sample to ensure it would come back conclusive. While having the ERA done, I met a nurse of Dr. Hoffman's, Lovely! She was indeed a Lovely lady. Her name really suited her, physically and personality wise. I can always count on IVF FL's great staff to help get through these crazy hectic processes. It was great speaking with her. She explained in her experience working with Dr. Hoffman, each and every time he performs an ERA, the patient gets pregnant on the next cycle they try which includes the adjustment of the protocol based on the ERA findings. That gave me lots of hope.

She herself was going through her own fertility woes. We exchanged numbers and have kept in contact since. As a medical professional, she said seeing patients get their success stories and living their dreams in an inspiration to her as well. So, in essence I gave her hope too.

The test was sent off to a lab in Spain, I believe, we expected the results in two weeks' time or so. One evening after settling in from work, the boys were playing on my phone, as per usual. They were at the age where they knew to answer the phone should it ring or at least find me or their dad so we could take the phone call. Needless to say, I was not expecting a call from Dr. Hoffman. I happened to be coming downstairs and I heard a voice on speaker and when I approached Kason, he handed me the phone and said, "Mommy he is calling back for you." It was Dr. Hoffman on the line. I was excited to hear from him. I must say I was a bit taken aback and though maybe something was wrong because it had not been the full allotted time yet for the results. We joked about him telling the boys not to hang up on him again, LOL. I said, "Yes Doc I'll have to remind them of who you are." ☺

Dr. Hoffman in his straight and to the point approach, immediately said "Ok Mar, we'll need an extra day of Progesterone!" I said, "Ohh OK, the results are back so quickly," and he laughed and said, "Yes, the lab I used expedited it for me. So, your lining was under receptive 24hrs, which means transferring on Day 5 was too premature. This test gets you down to the specific time frame. It's amazing." I replied, "Wow, this great news because at least we know something is different and a different approach can be used."

Dr. Hoffman said if I wanted we could start the next cycle or whenever I was ready.

ERA Done – 2nd Frozen Embryo Transfer Next

Of course, and as usual, I want to start now, smh. While I waited for my next menstrual cycle to start, the clinic put together my new protocol and got all the scripts ordered so I could have my meds. At this time, things because very hectic for our family and I had lots of work and filing deadlines to meet. So, although, I picked up all my meds, etc., we decided to take the next month, May/June off from starting the next cycle. That gave us time to get some things in order and focus on work, boys' year-end things, etc.

I decided to start with the late Jun/Jul cycle. I believe I started the protocol on 07.25.2017, the beginning of a menstrual cycle. At this point, my husband and I had planned a weekend away with the boys to Key West. Based on the protocol calendar, I was to begin Lupron and I think another med while on vacation. I took my injection with me to Key West to make sure I didn't miss a dose. I remember starting an injection on Sat, 08.05.2017, while away. It went well. My husband still didn't help with any of the injections, in case you were wondering, LOL. We had a lovely time that weekend with the twins. We really wanted to do something with them before the pregnancy. I just knew and felt confident it would work this time.

My FET, the actual embryo transfer, was scheduled for Fri, 08.11.2017. This was the date set after having been on the Progesterone for six days instead of five. It was another normal Friday. I was unable to get my pre-transfer acupuncture session in the night before. However, Dr. Duro agreed and wanted to do it for me the morning before I had to report to the clinic for my transfer. I had been doing my acupuncture religiously during this cycle as well as I did for the previous ones. I expressed the want to do my transfer after having acupuncture. Dr. Hoffman and the clinic are great supporters of this so they worked with the embryologists and timed the thawing of the embryos so I could make it in time. It worked out that the clinic was able to push me back to about 11:30 a.m. or so. So, my husband drove me to acupuncture at 9:30 or 10:00am and then we headed to and arrived at the clinic well in time.

We signed in at the front desk. The nurse had a nice embryo report waiting for me. She also provided me with a picture of the embryo after having been thawed. The baby was perfect! Not only by God's standards but also by embryo grading quality, if you want to explain it that way. I was then prepped and walked in to the operating room. It was Dr. Maxon this time who performed my embryo transfer. It was not on Dr. Hoffman's schedule that week, so he was unable to do it. Dr. Maxon was always good to us whenever I went in and had to work with him. He also had a very high successful implantation rate due to his ability to place the embryo in "perfect" position based on his measurements, the female's anatomy, etc. It was beautiful to watch. We were then given a picture of the embryo placement. It just looked like a white light in the center of the ultrasound picture.

Because it was a Friday, I was able to go home and just rest. They did not suggest bed rest but rather continue normal activities. This was definitely a different approach than my cycles back in 2011/2012. I was in bed, watched TV, hung with the boys, etc. I remember leaving the house the next day Saturday to go to the bank. In the midst of all of this, my identity was stolen. Yes!

Thus, I needed to get new accounts and the whole nine yards. While in the car with my husband either heading to or leaving the bank, I felt a sharp pain in my lower back. It was very pronounced and definitely startled me a bit. I said to myself, OK I am pregnant now that must be the embryo burrowing its way in getting nice and cozy.

The staff at the clinic helped calm me down because by Sunday, I was having fears that the embryo didn't survive the thaw. I even spoke to the lab and embryologist and they assured me the embryo was in great condition, and I should trust that nature will continue to take its course. I even texted Lovely and she assured me it was fine. Thank goodness for them. It's like even before you can find out for sure you're pregnant, your first sense as a mom is to worry and protect.

The Results Are In

The beta hCG test was scheduled for Monday, 08.21.2017. It was also the first day of school for the boys! My husband and I both took the day off. It became a tradition of ours to be off when we were anticipating the results of the pregnancy test. I went in early Monday morning after seeing the kids on to the bus. Everyone was feeling great about the results. They even asked me if I had tested early. I did, but didn't want to tell them.

I tested on Monday, 08.14.2017, just to see because when I went to brush my teeth that morning, I literally felt like I was going to throw up my entire intestines. That had never happened to me ever in life. I have heard other ladies experience this right before they tested positive but…. I bought a slew of Dollar Tree tests. I waited for those results and they seemed negative. I did not throw the test away, rather I put it in a drawer. Then Tuesday morning, I tested again and I think I saw what looked like a faint line. I started to sweat and freak out but didn't tell anyone. Wednesday, I tested and the line was darker. Needless to say I was cautiously optimistic. I wanted to think of a cute way to tell hubby. I just couldn't hold it in. I bought a card, a gift box and some baby ribbon and wrapped the tests up for him. Thursday evening, I told him to close his eyes because I had a gift. He looked confused and said, "Wait did I miss a special occasion, LOL?" I said no, you didn't but I have something for you. I pulled out my phone and started to record while I gave him the gift. He unwrapped the box, didn't even notice the baby ribbon, smh. He then opened the gift box and saw the sticks and he immediately smiled. 😊 He was like, "I thought you were going to wait for the official test; I knew you wouldn't be able to wait." It was a wonderful night and we were excited!

OK, so after having taken the blood test that morning at the clinic, I got home and just waited. I expected a call around 11:30 a.m. or so. Lovely was texting me explaining the results were not back yet because I missed the first lab pick up. It was probably because I went in for the test later because I wanted to see the kids on to the bus for the first day.

So, instead of being part of that 7 a.m. draw, I didn't get my test until closer to 8:30/9:00 or so.

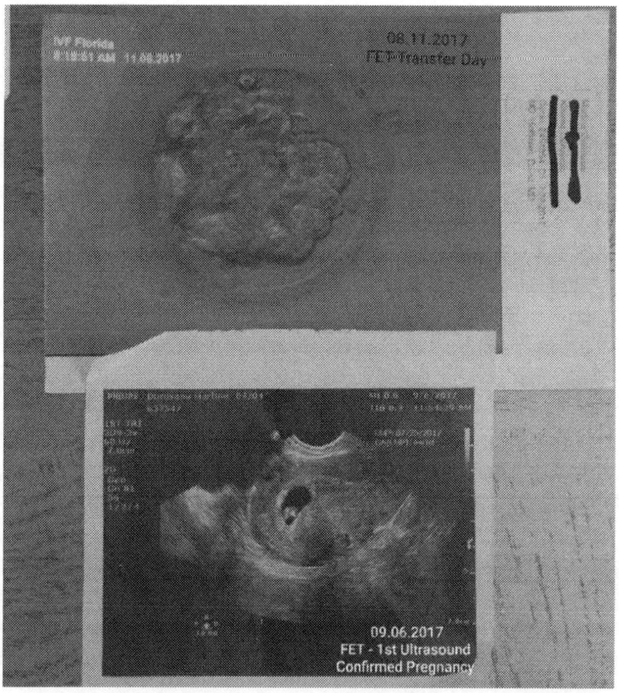

2017, IVF FL Embryology 6-day Blastocyst embryo for frozen transfer cycle

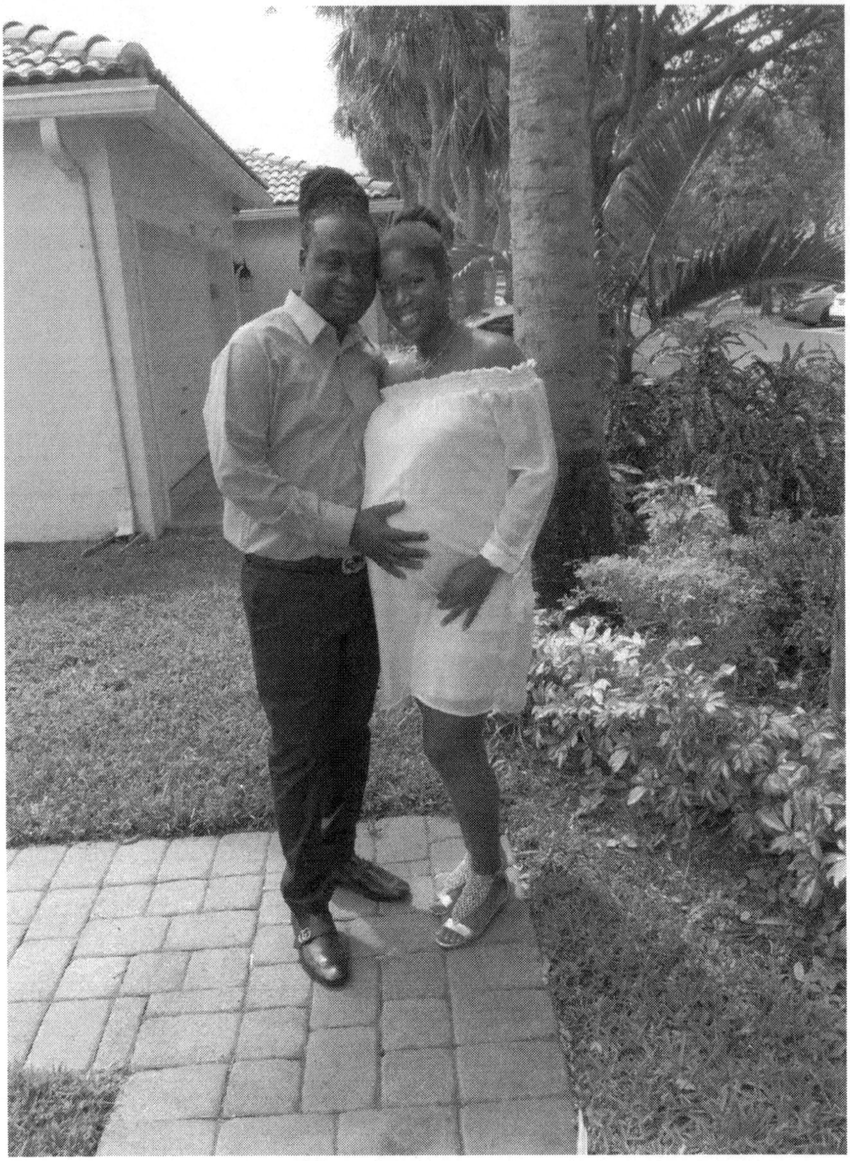

Easter Sunday, 04.01.18, two weeks later Kevens Benjamin was born on 04.18.18

We’re Pregnant!

Finally, I get the call around 2ish. Dr. H called me and after we answered the call, he said, “OK, kiddos, you did it again, you’re pregnant!” My beta is at 231 or 321 but it doubled and increased as it should as the days and weeks went by. This time around I had to be on the progesterone in oil (PIO) injections up until 10 weeks! It was tough because the needle was soooo big and the oil was thick so it took a while to go in. No worries though, I gladly poked myself daily for the next 6 weeks.

Dr. Hoffman is just great. He wanted to get me off to see the specialist OB/GYN asap. So he released me at eight weeks, and I scheduled my first OB visit at 9.5/10 weeks with Dr. Gene Burkett. Unfortunately, Dr. Yasin, the boys high-risk OB had retired. Dr. Hoffman gave me 3 suggestions and I loved Dr. Burkett.

I must say, the pregnancy continued on and went off without a hitch. It was a wonderful experience. I worked the entire time with no issues. At this time, I embarked on a new journey of teaching. I landed a position with Southern New Hampshire University as an adjunct accounting instructor. I taught online. The only main complaint I had was fatigue. As a new teacher and in my role at work, I was busy, busy, to say the least. I needed more energy to keep up with the mental work my brain had to focus on. Not sure how I got through it, but I did.

Because I had the TAC, I felt very secure in the pregnancy but also didn't want to overdo anything. We tried to have sex when I was almost out of the first trimester. I believe it was around 13 weeks or so. I have to tell you as soon as it was over both hubby and I looked at each and said, "Oh boy, we'll have to see how this is going to work." I started experiencing light pink spotting that wouldn't let up. The following Monday, I called Dr. Burkett and he told me not to wait and to come to see him in his Kendall office, I couldn't wait for his UM clinical day. He checked and everything looked OK. By then the spotting had stopped as well. I was 14 weeks on the ultrasound he had me do that day. It was wonderful to see the baby. He said to avoid any issues, no more pelvic stimulation until maybe after second trimester. We both gladly obliged.

Are We Team Pink or Team Blue?

That same week I had a genetic test done to ensure the baby was OK. I wanted to have a gender reveal as I hadn't had one before. My friend Mary Anne couldn't wait until the gender reveal to find out the results. She convinced me that someone needed to know in order to buy the reveal item so it might as well be her, LOL. So I gave Isis, Dr. Burkett's nurse, permission to disclose the sex of the baby to her via phone when she called. So, then my husband couldn't wait and wanted to know as well. So I told Mary Anne it was OK to tell him. So for many weeks only the two of them knew the sex of the baby. We had the soccer-themed gender reveal the weekend after Thanksgiving. It was the following Sunday. We wanted to wait for my mother-in-law to come to town because she was excited to confirm it was a girl. She leaves every August for Haiti and returns in Oct/Nov. She was so sure the baby was a girl that she came off the plane dressed in her pink dress. It was hilarious.

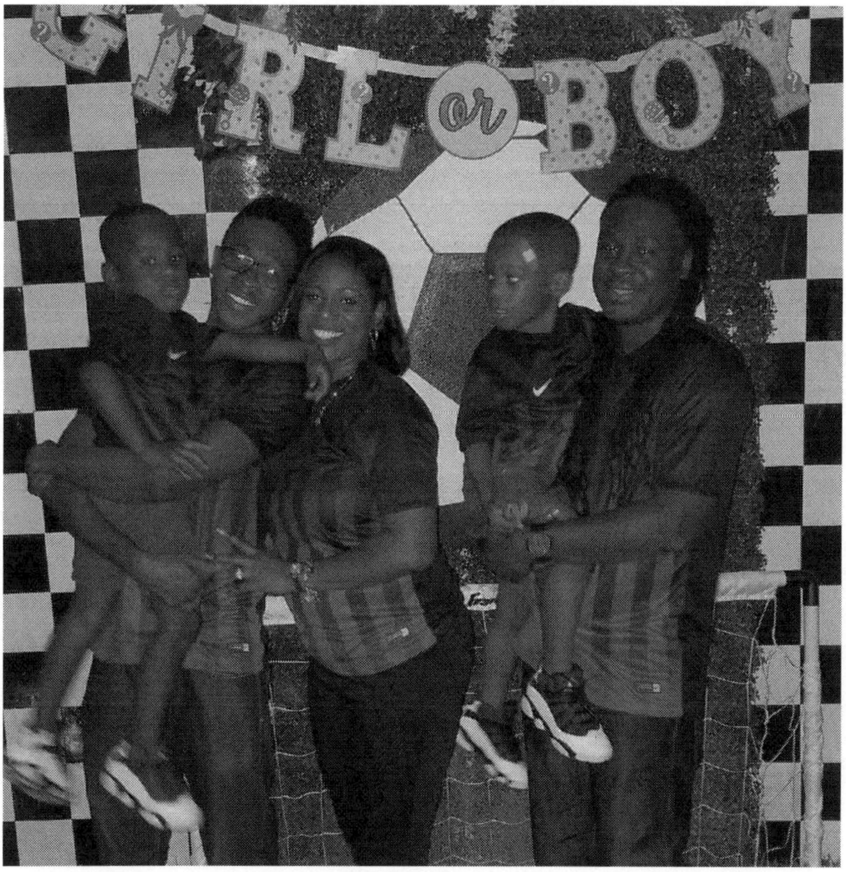

(Nov 2017 – appx 18wks pregnant: Soccer-Themed Gender Reveal in our backyard)

The gender reveal was a hit. I was soooo excited and nervous. I truly had no preference on the gender. However, no one believed me. They felt I secretly wanted a girl but wanted to protect my emotions in case it was a boy so that's why I wouldn't commit, smh. That was not the case. I was happy either way. I ordered balls with white powder for each of the boys to kick. However, it was bit too tough for the twins to actually penetrate them. So we didn't use those two. My bonus baby, Richard, kicked the first soccer ball. It got everyone going and riled up. We were surround by 48 family and friends, and they were excited.

Richard's ball had white powder so it definitely served as the test kick. My husband was up to kick the actual gender ball. He kicked the ball and BLUE powder spattered everywhere. It was great! He was soooo happy and ran around the backyard in excitement. It was a really fun day and great experience. I didn't think he'd react like that since he knew already but he was happy to finally let it out. We're having a BOY!

Let's Shower Him With Love

Everything else was just great and normal from there as it relates to the pregnancy. It was important to my husband for me to have a nice baby shower with an actual belly so we proceeded to work with my friend and planner Nerilanda w/HS Events (now Neri Events) to put the shower together. In January after the baby shower planning commenced, I had a heavy feeling in my vagina and a swollen right leg. Dr. Burkett had me immediately go to pregnancy ER and they did an ultrasound on my leg to ensure it wasn't a clot. It wasn't, so that was good. He also had them check my cervix via manual and ultrasound and it was closed and long. The TAC was doing its job. I guess because I had hit 23, almost 24, weeks the baby was getting bigger and put all his pressure on my lower right side, explaining the sudden symptoms I was having.

A month later, Feb 2018, my family and I were able to have our very first maternity photoshoot. I still can't believe it. It was the most perfect day. My planner and friend Neri helped put everything together for us. I picked out the looks I was going for and we went from there. One look would be me in a formal maternity blue dress with gold accessories. The guys wore black suspenders, white dress shirt, black dress pants and a gold bow tie. For the second look I wore a black bra, black Versace boxers, black pants and converse sneakers. The guys wore white A-shirts, black jeans and converse sneakers. My husband had white Versace boxers to compliment mine. So there was one formal and casual look. The pictures turned out beautifully. Our photographer Tony B and his team captured such memorable images of all of us. He even gave Kev abs, yes abs lol, on demand in a few of the pics as he requested! I think the pic with the abs were used as a snapchat filter for the shower. Great times! What made things even better was my friend taking the day off from work to accompany the family and me to the photoshoot and stayed the entire time. She was great in ensuring everything went off without a hitch and helping us get those wardrobe changes in. I was happy to have experienced that in my life like all the other pregnant mommies before me. 😊

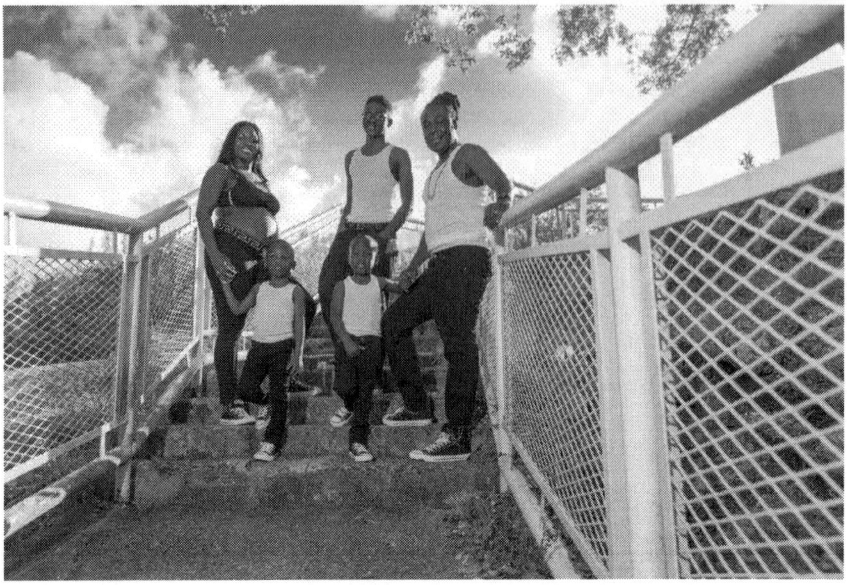

(Feb 2018 – Tony Barreau w/AVD Photography - Greynold's Park North Miami Beach, FL – Official Family/Maternity Photo, casual look!)

One week after the maternity shoot was the big day — my baby shower!!! I was so very excited. Again, Neri did a fantastic job at bringing my vision to life for the event. My husband was very impressed and I was glad because all I had to do was show up! I was already 31 weeks along. Everything was handled. My friends and family are always so gracious in helping us out during our events and the shower was no different. KB's shower reminded me of the twins' shower in that my friends handled everything. For those 2 showers, maybe the only times in my life, I let my crazy hands-on stressing go by the way side. My friends and family really outdid themselves and really showed out in supporting us and showing love to our family. I am extremely lucky and truly blessed. The baby got everything he could have needed and more. I was not expecting that at all. It was truly an overwhelming blessing.

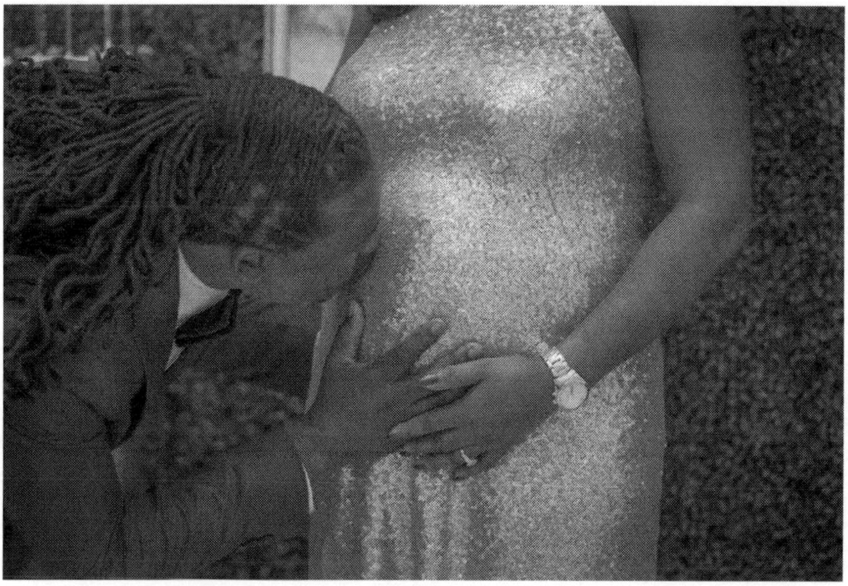

(Feb 2018 Walnut Creek Clubhouse, Pembroke Pines, FL – KB's Baby Shower – Pure Love)

Let's Talk about Sex

At this point in the pregnancy, it had been close to four months since my husband and I had tried to have sex. Remember the last time, at 13 weeks, there were some complications so we abstained since then. Because we were further along in the pregnancy and I was feeling well, we decided to try the night after the baby shower. I can tell you it was definitely an experience, LOL. My poor husband felt he didn't want to hurt me or the baby and I was just worried, smh. All in all, after the experience was over, of course I had another side effect. I felt like I couldn't stop shaking. I think they were contractions to be honest. It had been a while since my body was “worked up” so I figure I needed to calm down. Well, that didn’t happen. I felt those shakes for the entire night and into the next day. Needless to say, we didn’t do that anymore, LOL. I had an appointment later than week and explained to Dr. Burkett what happened. He said that yes, it must’ve been my body trying to orgasm and it couldn’t handle it. So he told us both to hold off since we waited so long already. He didn’t want for me to start having contractions and possibly rupture and deliver because of having sex. So we gladly obliged.

I must say during this entire fertility journey we learned so much about what it means to have a true connection. That connection doesn’t always have be a physical one. As a married couple who didn’t have kids for a long time during the marriage, all of our time was spent together. Much of this together time involved lots and lots of sex. I mean, what else was there to do while we waited? Having that dynamic in the relationship really set the tone for what was to be expected when it came to sex.

Unfortunately, even if you come to expect certain things, the couple has to evolve and compromise when extenuating circumstances present themselves causing the need to deviate from the norm. We had been trying to get pregnant, medically, since 2003. We finally became pregnant in 2011 and reached the end of our fertility journey in 2018. During those 15 years, there were lots of times where we experienced prolonged timeframes of no sex. I have to say that during my younger years, when in my 20s, it was difficult to abstain. As I got older in my 30s, it wasn’t an issue for me. I was more focused on the end goal than anything else.

Now when it came to my husband, that is a different story. Not being able to engage in sexual activity for him was definitely a significant issue. I guess it's safe to say men love sex! I mean they rarely ever get tired of it. In our case, we averaged sex maybe 3 times a week, sometimes 4. It just depends on the week of the month. I'm sure my husband could have done it more often but that was our normal average and it was consistent so it was OK and worked.

Sex During 1st Pregnancy

Before we knew I had a cervix issue, we had sex regularly during my first pregnancy with Angel. Once we found out there was an issue and I needed surgery, there was no sex until six weeks after I delivered. So that meant close to three months of no sex for him. That was the first and longest time we'd gone without having sex. When I was ready to engage in activity again, it was hard for my husband because I would start crying. I had intermittent bursts of unexplained emotional setbacks after losing Angel. He felt bad and didn't know how to help me. So when I cried during sex, he felt confused, helpless, and saddened.

No Sex During Twin Pregnancy

During our second pregnancy with the twins, there was almost no sex at all. During the IVF cycle, once you start stimulation medications, Dr. Hoffman advised against sex and if we did it, it had to be protected. Once I became pregnant from the cycle, there was still no sex. They did not want to mess with anything in my pelvic region while the embryos were trying really burrow in to the lining. That took us to about the mid first trimester. After those 10–12 weeks we may have had sex once. Then sex was off the table again when I had the preventative cerclage put in at about 12 weeks or so with the twins. Dr. Yasin cautioned against sex, rather pelvic rest. So nothing in or out of the vaginal area. So during the twins' pregnancy, we can say there was no penetration going on. The good thing is we found other ways to meet the needs but it couldn't involve too much stimulation so my body wouldn't start to contract. Needless to say, things were really tricky in the sex arena during that pregnancy.

No Sex and More No Sex

During the last pregnancy, we tried twice but to no avail. So that was maybe the fifth stint of long periods with no sex. Let's not forget the cycle that resulted in miscarriage, then the failed third IVF cycle before I got pregnant the last time. Sex is not on the radar really when cycling. Sometimes the doctors caution against it. Sometimes, the hormones cause us women to not even want it. Oftentimes, while cycling your body causes you varying degrees of discomfort and pain. Thus, physically sex would be hard to even get through. Even though the men would probably still want to have sex, when they see all the happenstance that the medicated cycle brings, they too back off, just a little bit.

Sex From His View

All in all, we've had many prolonged periods of not being able to have sex. To be honest, I felt bad as though it was my fault for not being able to have a baby normally and have sex while pregnant like normal women and couples do. I asked my husband what his take was on this topic. Kev smiled and said, "Well, I can tell you there was lots of hand action during those times." I laughed and said what, I didn't know that. He explained oh yeah, that's what I had to do so it wasn't a problem. I asked if he felt bad because I felt like I let him down. He explained, after the first pregnancy he was freaked out. He learned a lot about my cervix and said he didn't want to jeopardize our chances of having kids because he couldn't wait. He said, "It was a huge sacrifice but I'd do it again." He quoted an old Haitian saying that says, "Better to take the long, slow bumpy road and arrive safely than to rush and lose your way." It's not a literal translation but definitely close and along those lines. My husband is definitely a trooper!

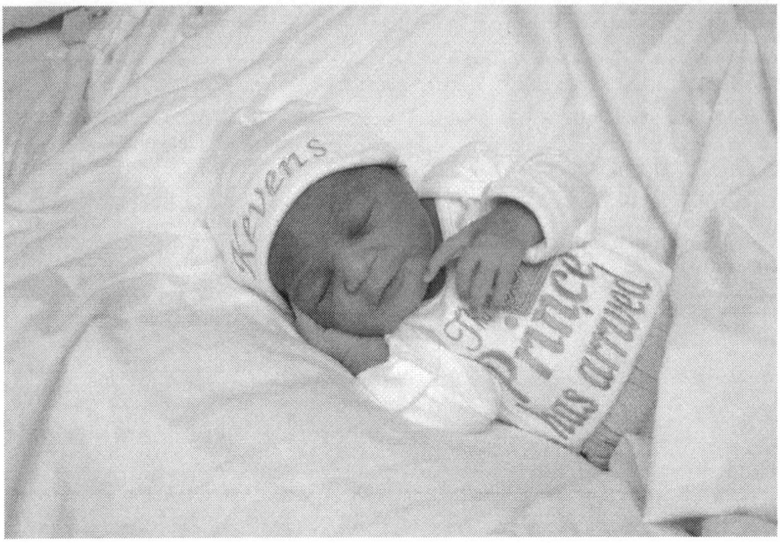

(Apr 2018 Holtz Children's at Jackson Memorial Hospital, Miami, FL, Kevens Benjamin is born!)

The Aftermath

I delivered our healthy 7lbs 13oz, 21.5 inches long beautiful baby boy on my scheduled C-section date of 04.18.2018 at 38+1 weeks. When you have a TAC, the fear of rupturing is great so you don't really make it to your actual due date, which was 05.01.2018 for me. It was perfect! Out came Kevens Benjamin (KB) into our world. I never liked the idea of a Jr so we reached a compromise. The baby would be named after my husband but we'd call him by his initials. We eventually settled on Benjamin because it means Beloved. So, our KB is indeed beloved and is the newest bright light of our family.

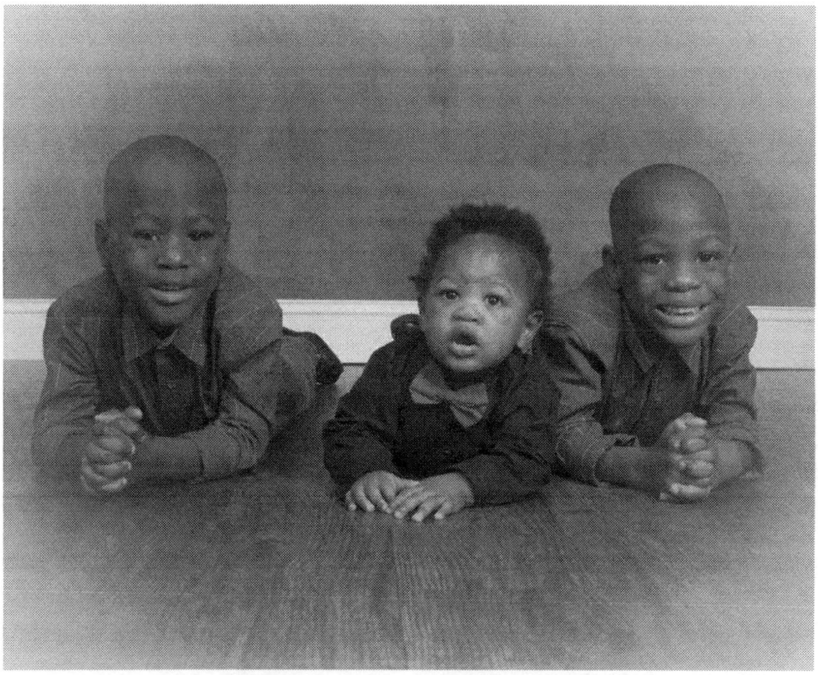

(Jan 2019 JC Penney @ Aventura, FL, KB is 9 months and the twins are 6)

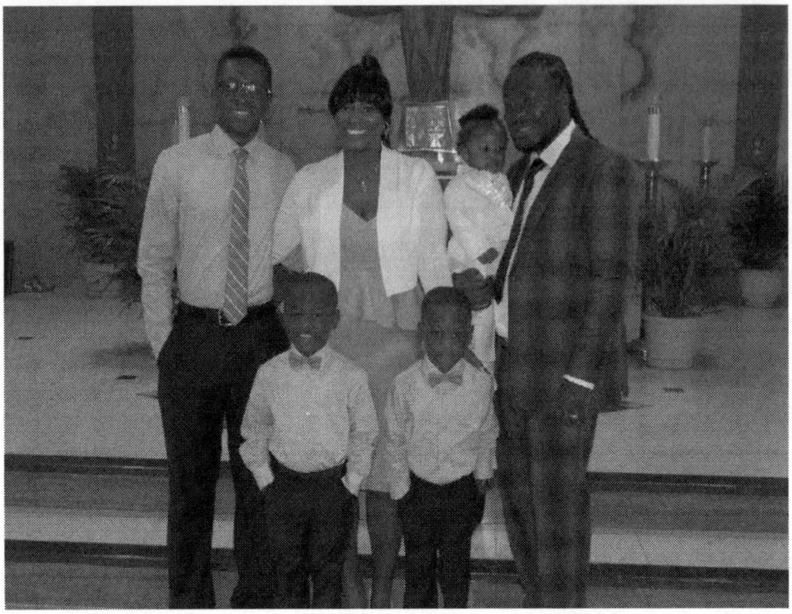

(Apr 2019 Church of the Visitation of the Blessed Virgin Mary, Miami, FL – KB's Baptism)

Life with three little boys now is just perfect or perfect for us. My husband is beyond excited to have all these boys. The twins took really well to their little brother. We were worried they'd be jealous or feel left out. That was not the case at all. KB bought his brothers big brother gifts that he presented to them when he was born. They were very happy that the baby thought about them and bought them a gift. They were amazed he knew exactly what they liked. They made my heart smile when they opened their gifts at the hospital. They came to see KB in the hospital Friday evening. I had the baby on Wednesday and as to not interrupt their daily routine with school, etc., we waited until Friday to have them visit. Even Rich received a big brother gift.

I shared this story of the gifts because all of the boys settled well into their roles as big brothers. They do their best to help, protect and love each other. As there is a 17-year age difference between Richard and the twins, there is a 5 ½ year age gap between the twins and KB. It's such a beautiful dynamic between all of them.

The experience I had after delivering KB was significantly different than any of the other postpartum delivery experiences. This time everyone came to visit and I actually had my beautifully healthy baby in my room with me. It was truly a family affair. Everyone visited and we just enjoyed the experience. It reminded me of all the other visits we'd make to see anyone else in our family or friends who had delivered babies. It was joyous. Although, there was now no longer a nursery for the babies to go to. Yep, they were in that room with mommy, for bonding, from the moment you're out of recovery, LOL. The great thing is that my sister was there every day to help me and to keep the baby while I tried to rest. It was just great. I have to tell you that it was a kind of weirdly proud moment to have my oldest niece, Beatrice, be there with me, now as an adult, to also help me during that recovery time. She was in school but was also a nurse. So guess who gave me my first bath/shower after having the baby, yep it was her. My baby niece who I helped raised like my own (I was 13 when she was born) was now taking care of me. It was a very proud and fulfilling experience and a beautiful memory I will always have, even though it came with her seeing me with the oversized boobs, and soiled chucks and mesh panties and the ever so popular sitz bottle process. I felt like a new woman after that bath, lol.

My husband and I have finally been able to make our way back to each other again. The kids are getting older. Richard is 25, Kason and Kamden are 8 and KB is almost 3. Things were definitely tough for me and how I viewed our relationship after the twins. That is and will be a whole separate writing of its own. All in all, we grew a lot as a couple and learned from the experiences we had with each other after the twins. We didn't want to repeat some of those same unsettling things. This experience was extremely different in that big Kev was 110% hands-on and dedicated to helping care for KB. He did everything! It's almost like I just carried and delivered him and that's it. Obviously there was a lot that I, as mom, had to do but he was a significant help with the baby and still is. I definitely found the post-baby experience this time around with KB was in great contrast of the post-baby experience with the twins. For that I am thankful. He kept the promise he made to me after agreeing to try again – that this time it would be different, and it was. Big Kev keeps thanking me almost daily for agreeing to be with him and for giving him a beautiful family. We go to church each week as the boys started CCD and are slated to receive their first communion in May 2021. Things got a bit interesting for us while having to be quarantined during corona virus. The boys have also adapted to virtual school as a result and now face-to-face instruction.

In spite of everything we've been through to start our family, we would do it again in a heartbeat. I am so thankful and feel blessed and lucky to have the support and guidance from the Lord and everyone he's put on our path to obtaining our joy. I often wonder what I would have done if our story wasn't written this way. When I have those thoughts, I immediately venture away from them because I don't want to doubt Him. I just felt deep down inside I'd be a mom, one way or another. Not only did I have a desire, I worked hard to obtain it with both divine and medical intervention. As such, it was not easy and I do not regret any part of my journey.

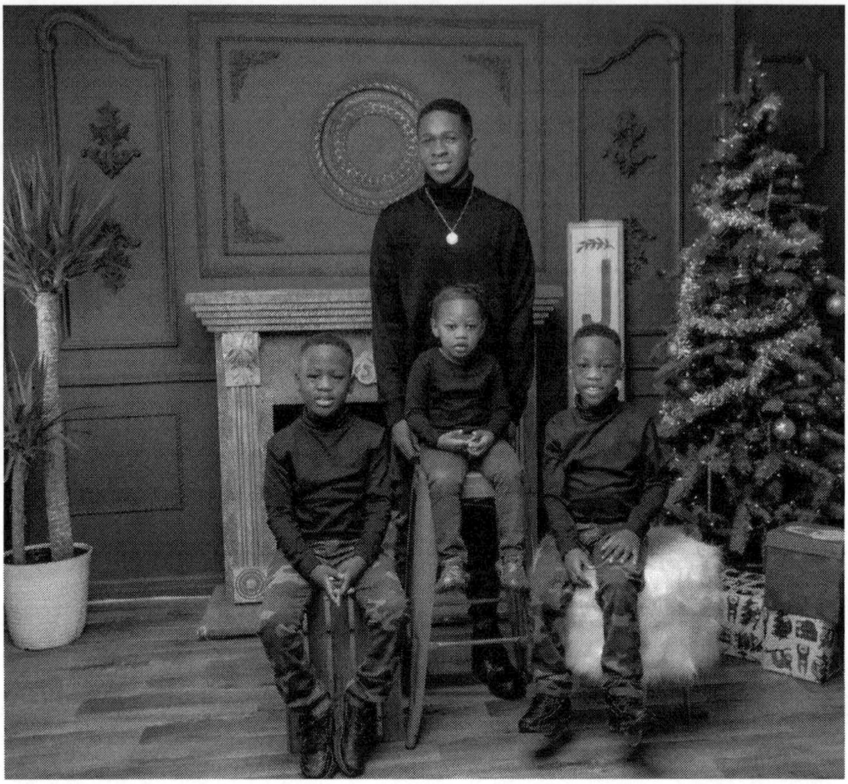

(Dec 2020 Johnny Luc w/ RedLight Photography, Lauderhill, FL, Holiday Shoot – 4 Duroseau Princes)

Final Lessons from the Journey

As much as I have faith, I also know that Faith Without Works is dead. Thus, that was a great part of my motivation to keep going! Although I wasn't quite sure of how exactly I'd obtain my family, I just knew one day I'd have one. God made a promise to me and I trusted and believed and worked while I waited for him to fulfill that promise.

Having gone through so much over the years as it relates to starting a family, some important things stand out for me to share with others who may be going through the same or a similar situation. Be encouraged and keep the faith! One's mindset is almost more than half the battle in anything we face. If you go into any endeavor thinking you won't finish or thinking it won't work out, chances are it may not. This is partly because of the non-positive vibes being put in to the atmosphere. It's easier said than done but try and find the positive in every situation. The affect that has on your psyche will really make an impact.

It is also important to live through the tough times. There is never a promise that everything you want will come fast and easily. I don't think that's even possible. Some couples' journeys may not be all traumatic but be open to knowing in the event something doesn't go as planned, it's OK to just experience it. If you try to ignore it or push through it without acknowledging it or admitting how it makes you feel or impacted you, you will not be able to heal properly. Healing comes in many forms. There is no right or wrong way to heal. Many people will have an opinion but it is ultimately up to you. Take advantage of the many resources available to help. Trusted family members, friends or spiritual leader, support groups, therapy or counseling, yoga, and meditation are just some of the avenues you can explore.

Part of this journey involves finding the right set of medical professionals. Don't feel like you have to be stuck with a particular clinic or doctor. Having faith also involves trusting the people employed to help you achieve your dreams. So, if you don't trust or feel confident in the process or people, it will impact you and your chances of success as well. Build a rapport with your medical team and also educate yourself as much as possible. That way everyone is on the same page.

My husband often says time and time again to me, "Marline, we've been through a lot. I am happy we didn't give up. We've been through hell and back but we have a beautiful end result to show for it. Our family is our prize." He strongly feels that if there's even a glimmer of hope, look past the tough times and envision the win on the other side in an effort to get through. Although our relationship dynamics changed a bit after the birth of the twins, my husband's support and empathy for me during all the trying times of our fertility journey never faltered. He made it clear and still does that we are in this together. It is important to have the unconditional support of your partner in order to succeed. Not having a united front or solid partnership will inevitably make your fertility journey even more complicated to say the least.

Although my family's fertility journey resulted in the birth of our biological children, many other families are formed via other means. This includes surrogacy via gestational carrier, donor eggs, donor sperm, and adoption. How and when does a couple decide which method to employ? How and when do they determine when it's time to move on to other means? Those are unequivocally loaded questions that don't have a right or wrong answer. Each family is unique. They must find their own happy medium. One that satisfies their wishes and outcome to the best of their goal intentions for their family.

It Happened By 30 but...

There's something humbling about having a plan. Although we're conditioned to think things through, plan things out and have a contingency in place, the results do not always match up. The idea of not having everything work out in the manner in which you intended can and will throw you for a loop. Sometimes the plan works out as intended and for the best. Other times the plan results in an outcome that just isn't as good.

In my case, the thought of it happening by 30 served more as a faith-filled manifestation of what I wanted for my life. I knew I had to work hard and do my part, but I also kept believing and knew it would happen.

Consequently, the plan worked out but not in the way I ever imagined it would. Just as fast as my dream came true by 30, it was quickly taken away from me at 30. (It's funny because) from a faith standpoint, I questioned why God would let this happen? He granted my wish just to take it away? Why?

It took me a long time to deal with all the fall out of emotions that centered around that horrible experience I had. I don't think I ever actually received the answer to my question. However, He and I have ongoing conversations all the time and ultimately I know He is looking out for my and my family's best interest. I find ultimate comfort in knowing that. My faith is and will continue to be the foundation I stand on.

"Blessed is she who believed..."

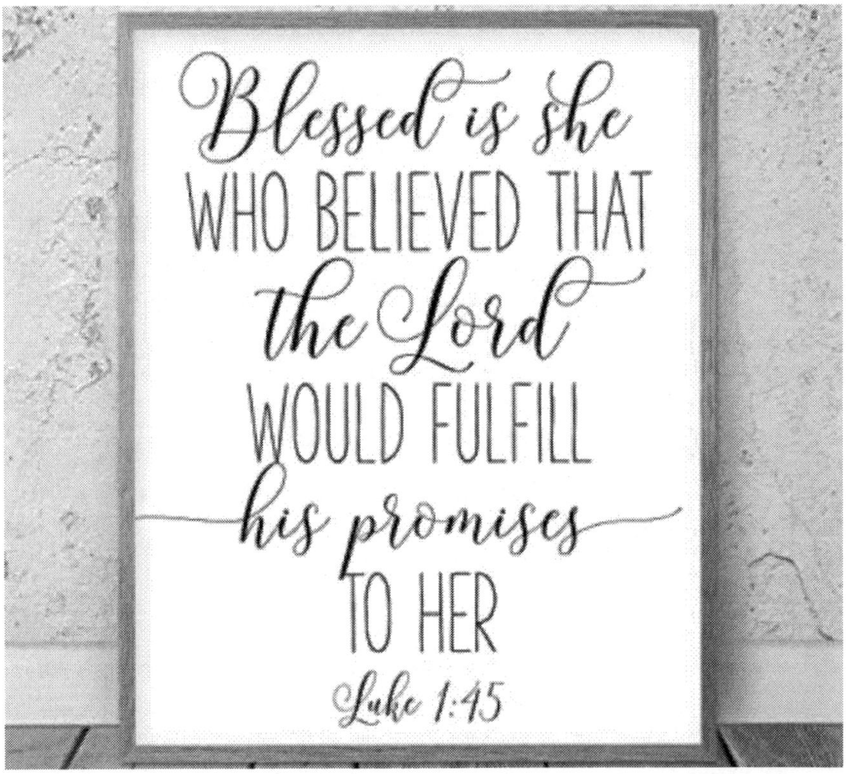

(One of my favorite faith reminders: Luke 1:45 – "Blessed is She Who Believed That the Lord Would Fulfill His Promise to Her")

My quest to have more children has ended. I hope sharing my experience will encourage others or serve as an example as families embark on the journey to have a family of their own.
To say we've been blessed is an understatement!

1 Samuel 1:27 For this child I prayed, and the LORD has granted me my petition that I made to him.

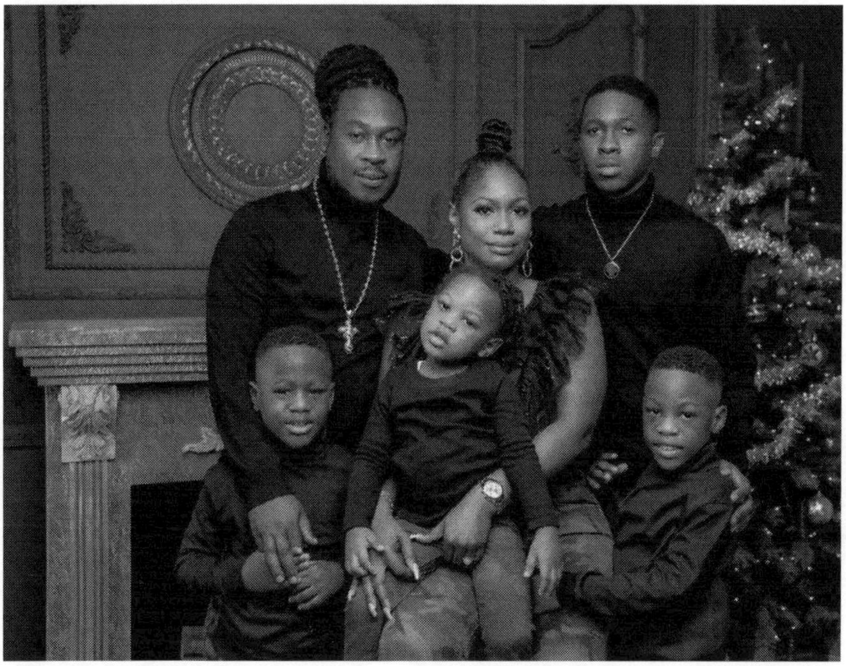

(Dec 2020 Johnny Luc w/RedLight Photography, Lauderhill, FL)

We Prayed, We Sacrificed, We Triumphed

Made in the USA
Monee, IL
05 November 2026

67811028R00139